Student Nurses' Guide to Professional Practice and Development

Edited by

Jane E Schober RGN, DipN Ed, DipN (Lond), RCNT, RNT, MN
Principal Lecturer, School of Nursing and Midwifery,
De Montfort University, Leicester, UK

Carol Ash RN, HV, DipN (Lond), DipN Ed, RCNT, RNT, B Ed (Hons), MBA
Independent Nurse Education Consultant
Formerly Senior Lecturer, School of Nursing and Midwifery,
De Montfort University, Leicester, UK

Hodder Arnold

A MEMBER OF THE HODDER HEADLINE GROUP
LONDON

First published in Great Britain in 2006 by
Hodder Education, a member of the Hodder Headline Group,
338 Euston Road, London NW1 3BH

http://www.hoddereducation.com

Distributed in the United States of America by
Oxford University Press Inc.,
198 Madison Avenue, New York, NY 10016
Oxford is a registered trademark of Oxford University Press

Whilst the advice and information in this book are believed to be true and
accurate at the date of going to press, neither the author[s] nor the publisher
can accept any legal responsibility or liability for any errors or omissions
that may be made. In particular, (but without limiting the generality of the
preceding disclaimer) every effort has been made to check drug dosages;
however it is still possible that errors have been missed. Furthermore,
dosage schedules are constantly being revised and new side-effects
recognized. For these reasons the reader is strongly urged to consult the
drug companies' printed instructions before administering any of the drugs
recommended in this book.

British Library Cataloguing in Publication Data
A catalogue record for this book is available from the British Library

Library of Congress Cataloging-in-Publication Data
A catalog record for this book is available from the Library of Congress

ISBN-10   0 340 75970 4
ISBN-13   978 0 340 75970 7

1 2 3 4 5 6 7 8 9 10

Commissioning Editor: Clare Christian
Project Editor: Heather Smith/Clare Patterson
Production Controller: Jane Lawrence
Cover Design: Georgina Hewitt

Typeset in 9.5/12 Berling Roman by Charon Tec Pvt. Ltd, Chennai, India
www.charontec.com
Printed and bound in Great Britain by Martins The Printers, Berwick-upon-Tweed.

What do you think about this book? Or any other Hodder Arnold title?
Please send your comments to www.hoddereducation.com

Student Nurses' Guide to Professional Practice and Development

Contents

327230

Appendices

List of Contributors

Carol Ash RN, HV, DipN (Lond), DipN Ed, RCNT, RNT, B Ed (Hons), MBA
Independent Nurse Education Consultant, formerly Senior Lecturer, School of Nursing and Midwifery, De Montfort University, Leicester, UK

Veronica Bishop PhD, MPhil, RGN, FRSA
Editor, *Nursing Times Research* and Professor of Nursing, School of Nursing and Midwifery, De Montfort University, Leicester, UK

Penny Harrison MA, BSc (Hons), RGN, ENB 100, Cert Ed
Senior Lecturer, School of Nursing and Midwifery, De Montfort University, Leicester, UK

Kevin Power MA, BA (Hons), RSCN, RGN, DipN (Lond), Cert Ed
Principal Lecturer, School of Nursing and Midwifery, De Montfort University, Leicester, UK

Nick Salter RGN, DipN (Lond), Cert Ed (Adults), BSc (Hons), MA, LTM
Senior Lecturer, School of Nursing and Midwifery, De Montfort University, Leicester, UK

Jane E Schober RGN, DipN Ed, DipN (Lond), RCNT, RNT, MN
Principal Lecturer, School of Nursing and Midwifery, De Montfort University, Leicester, UK

Ben Thomas MSc, BSc (Hons), DipN (Lond), RGN, RMN, RNT, CertHE, FRCN
Director of Nursing and Organisational Development, Somerset Partnership NHS and Social Care Trust, and Principal Lecturer, University of Plymouth, Plymouth, UK. Currently on secondment as Chief Nurse, St Vincent's Mental Health Service, Melbourne, Australia

Robert Tunmore MA, DGDip (Ed), BSc (Hons), RGN, RMN, RNT
Nursing Officer, Communications, Department of Health
Formerly Academic Co-ordinator and Principal Lecturer, University of Plymouth, Plymouth, UK

Maureen Turner RNMH, RNM, RNT, DipN (Lond) A&B, MA
Principal Lecturer, School of Nursing and Midwifery, De Montfort University, Leicester, UK

Acknowledgements

With thanks to the Nursing and Midwifery Council for their permission to reproduce the material in Appendices 1–3, and to the Sainsbury Centre for Mental Health for permission to reproduce *A Framework for Capable Practice* in Appendix 4.

Introduction and How to Use This Book

Nursing is one of the most challenging and diverse careers available to you. Though demanding, those who have a commitment to care for and support those who have health and nursing needs will find a vast range of career opportunities, following successful completion of a pre-registration nursing course.

If you want to know about a career in nursing, professional requirements and practice, entry into nursing courses and the branch programmes, this is the book for you. This book is for anyone considering or embarking on a nursing career. It is a valuable resource for student nurses, nursing cadets, and health care assistants considering a nursing course. It contains a wealth of information about nursing as a career, being a student nurse, the four branches of nursing, support networks for students and key aspects of professional development for students preparing to register as a qualified nurse. It is a detailed introduction to the professional issues relating to career and professional development for student nurses. It will also provide anyone considering a nursing career with information about nursing courses and the range of practice opportunities that exist in the United Kingdom.

Each chapter is written by an experienced nurse and author, an expert in the chosen field. Each chapter contains an introduction summarizing the main content, reflective exercises to invite you to apply key issues to your own experiences, and detailed references and further reading options to support the main issues. Most chapters contain a glossary to explain key terminology and there are many useful addresses and websites included to facilitate your need for further information and support.

The inclusion of three appendices containing Nursing and Midwifery Council information which is pertinent to student nurses, professional requirements and professional development, is referred to throughout the chapters and is a convenient resource for the reader.

We hope that you find this book a useful resource as you pursue your nursing career.

Jane E Schober
Carol Ash

Embarking On a Career in Nursing

Jane E Schober

INTRODUCTION

Most of us will need a nurse at some point in our lives. By embarking on a career in nursing, you are entering a profession with a long history and a reputation for having the care of others at its heart. The motivation to care for others in various states of mental, physical and emotional health is characteristic of many applicants to nursing courses. Indeed, caring has been viewed as the fundamental value of nursing, and as such implies that nurses are prepared to express skilled, compassionate care for those who require it. The complexity of nursing is evident as any interaction, nursing and health care activity will be influenced by the needs and individuality of those requiring a service.

Currently courses are available with branch programmes in all or some of the four branches of nursing, preparing students to register as an adult, children's, learning disability or mental health nurse. In addition, there is a wide range of roles for qualified nurses: thus the employment opportunities are great, making nursing a potentially life-long career. This chapter aims to provide an overview of the potential of nursing as a career and includes the following sections:

- Introduction to nursing
- Becoming a nurse: applying for a course in nursing
- Professional issues: preparing to gain your licence to practise nursing
- Your nursing course.

INTRODUCTION TO NURSING

There are many challenges facing nurses today. The health and social care systems in the UK aim to provide services for the population that support and promote health, prevent illness and provide treatment and care for patients, clients, carers, families and communities. This is a complex service that is influenced by the demands on national and local resources, health policies, nursing policies and health care priorities. Nurses form the largest proportion of the National Health Service (NHS) workforce and are also present in large numbers in the independent and voluntary health care sectors. As such, they are an essential part of how health and nursing care is planned, organized and managed.

Raised public expectation and understanding of health care issues places increasing demands on health care professionals to provide quality care that is personalized. The *NHS Improvement Plan* (Department of Health (DoH), 2004) explains the NHS priorities between now and 2008. Three priorities are summarized as follows:

- 'putting patients and service users first through more personalized care
- a focus on the whole of health and well-being, not only illness; and
- further devolution of decision-making to local organisations' (DoH, 2005).

This builds on *The NHS Plan* (DoH, 2000) which is a 10-year programme to reform key aspects of the NHS. It marked the start of the most comprehensive shake up of the NHS since it came into being in 1948. It included strategies to personalize the service, targets to reduce waiting times for treatment, invest in new facilities and services, increase the number of consultants and nurses and provide opportunities for staff development. National standards for health care were established including the National Institute for Health and Clinical Excellence (NICE), which makes recommendations about treatments, and National Service Frameworks, which makes recommendations about standards of care for care groups (see Useful websites at the end of the chapter).

Nurses are in the front line of health care delivery. They may work independently, in teams and in a range of health and social care settings. It is a challenge to summarize the essence of nursing, but it is true to suggest that the nature of the needs of patients and clients demands that nurses use their skills to adapt to them in a way that promotes their well-being, healing and care in a respectful way. The Royal College of Nursing (RCN) suggests that the primary purpose of nursing is to:

> provide holistic health and health care for patients, families, carers and communities. Registered nurses are responsible for maintaining all aspects of the health environment so that it is conducive to improving health, facilitating recovery from illness or rehabilitation, and where appropriate, achieving a dignified death.

(RCN, 2004, p. 4)

Reflective activity

From this introduction, aim to write your definition of nursing. Try to express your values and priorities about what you think nursing represents for those needing care.

Compare your definition with the following RCN definition which states:

> The use of clinical judgement in the provision of care to enable people to improve, maintain, or recover health, to cope with health problems, and to achieve the best possible quality of life, whatever their disease or disability, until death.

(RCN, 2004, p. 4)

Another definition, long respected and referred to by nurses, was given by Virginia Henderson (1966):

> The unique function of the nurse is to assist the individual, sick or well, in the performance of those activities contributing to health or its recovery (or to a peaceful death) that he would perform unaided if he had the recovery strength, will or knowledge. And to do this in

such a way as to help him gain independence as rapidly as possible.

Nursing is about helping, supporting and intervening to care for and promote the health of those who need interventions in a skilled, professional way. Being sensitive, kind, communicative, non-judgemental and respectful to the individuality of the person concerned is essential. An awareness of and sensitivity to individual cultures, religions and lifestyles supports this process.

Students who embark on a nursing career face exciting challenges. The following sections provide information to support this process.

BECOMING A NURSE: APPLYING FOR A COURSE IN NURSING

Getting started

There are over 60 centres in higher education institutions (HEIs) and colleges in the UK offering nursing courses. Choosing a course, the branch programme and whether to opt for a degree or diploma course (in England only) will be influenced by:

- your academic qualifications
- where you plan to undertake the course
- your chosen branch programme
- your social circumstances and family commitments
- your ability to travel or commute
- your financial circumstances
- your long-term career goals (if you know them).

Careful consideration of these factors along with detailed fact-finding about the available courses is essential. Student numbers on the course, available accommodation, resources and facilities for students and how the structure of the course and the timetable may influence your needs are essential to your planning.

Most nursing courses are full time. They are three years in length with a 45-week academic year spread over three semesters. Fifty per cent of the course timetable is theoretical and based in the university or college, the other fifty per cent is in practice, to gain practice-based experience. Therefore you are expected to adapt to learning in two quite contrasting arenas. When in practice, the student nurse usually follows the duty rotas of the nurses in that ward or unit, especially of those who are assigned to the student's support and learning experiences. Shift work and some night duty will be necessary for these experiences. So unlike many university students, student nurses are subject to:

- academic and educational objectives relating to course work
- practice placement objectives to fulfil practice standards
- professional development objectives expected of student nurses.

Course information

Information about HEIs and colleges are available from their own websites, professional bodies, e.g. the Nursing and Midwifery Council (NMC), the Universities and Colleges Admissions Service (UCAS) and the Nursing and Midwifery Admission Service (NMAS) (see Useful websites below). Most HEIs offer summer schools, open days and taster courses which you can attend to find out more about the university and the courses of interest. Details of these are advertised on the HEI website.

Academic entry requirements

Usually the MINIMUM academic entry requirements for pre-registration nursing courses are five GCSEs at C grade or above that include English language and a science subject or equivalent.

A detailed range of qualifications equates with these and information about these may be obtained from either UCAS or NMAS. There are pre-registration nursing courses in all the countries in the UK. Many HEIs offer pre-registration courses: 50 in England, seven in Scotland, three in Northern Ireland (including the Open University) and six in Wales. Many centres offer courses in all branches of nursing, namely:

- Adult nursing
- Children's nursing
- Learning disability nursing
- Mental health nursing.

The courses can be at degree or diploma level.

Degree courses

All the countries in the UK offer full time degree-level courses which are 3 or 4 years in length. In addition, there are a few sandwich or shortened courses for graduates. However, many degree and some diploma courses do not offer all the branch programme options.

Entry to these courses depends on meeting the HEI entry requirements. Applicants (except those with access courses) must have a minimum of five GCSEs at grade C or above or equivalent, to include, English language, mathematics and at least one science subject. In addition, degree-course applicants would be expected to achieve additional academic qualifications, the details of which are available through UCAS (see Useful websites below) and the HEIs.

Diploma courses

In England, most HEIs offer degree and diploma level courses. Diploma courses are usually full time for 3 years though there are some part-time courses available. As with degree courses, some centres do not offer all the branch options. Applicants must demonstrate evidence of numeracy and literacy skills and good character, details of which are available from NMAS (see Useful websites below).   CRB -

Other routes for entering diploma and degree courses – flexible entry opportunities

Foundation degrees

These are in their early stages but may facilitate entry to year 2 of a nursing course.

Access to higher education courses

If you do not have GCSEs or other academic qualifications equivalent to the minimum entry requirements, you can take an access course. This is a course to Access Higher Education and for nursing, is 1 year full time or two years part time.

Nursing cadet schemes

In England, there are over 60 nursing cadet schemes that allow you to achieve a National Vocational Qualification at level 3 (NVQ 3) if you do not have other academic qualifications. This facilitates access to the diploma courses.

Secondments

If you are employed as a health care assistant (HCA) within the NHS, there may be an opportunity for you to be seconded onto a course. This will mean that your salary will continue being paid and there is an expectation that you will return to the same practice area after the course, although this is not essential.

Other entry requirements

As well as fulfilling academic entry requirements, you also need to be 17-and-a-half years of age on the day the course starts and at least 16 years when you apply. Each HEI has additional entry requirements which include:

- health screening
- Criminal Records Bureau (CRB) checks.

The HEI may also require:

- evidence of previous relevant caring experience
- attendance at interview
- academic qualifications additional to the minimum already described, especially for degree courses.

Informal visit

Visiting a prospective university or college is essential. Aim to talk to current students if you can. Explore the campus and facilities such as the library and student union. Notice boards may reveal how active some of the clubs and support facilities are. Consider your accommodation needs, and if you are not familiar with the campus or area where the course is based, it is useful to explore the accommodation on offer as well as transport facilities, especially if placements are not geographically near to the campus.

Summary

- Carefully examine your motives for applying for a nursing course.
- There are different routes for accessing nursing courses in the UK.
- Ensure you have detailed knowledge about your chosen course, HEI and branch programme.
- Nursing courses demand that you adapt to learning during practice placements, produce the required academic work and assignments and develop professionally.

Being a student nurse

Student nurses often express a mix of excitement and apprehension, enthusiasm and reservation at what may lie ahead. Nursing courses are busy, demanding, challenging and dynamic. The variety of practice experiences along with the educational demands suggest that you need to be organized, because it is also important to enjoy university life and to take advantage of meeting other students as well as working to your full potential during the course.

Several demands that face all students will also impact on student nurses. Many have come away from home for the first time and home sickness is very real for a lot of students (see Chapter 8). Making ends meet is a common stress and depending on whether you are following a degree or a diploma course, the financial arrangements will differ. Details of financial support are available through HEIs and the Department of Health (DoH, 2003). Adapting to the course, fellow students and new environments may be challenging. Your main sources of support during the course will be the following:

Course leader and lecturers: Lecturers are responsible for organizing the course, providing detailed information, guidance and support. Each part of the course or module will have a leader and a team of lecturers who teach, assess, provide resource material and feedback about your course work and overall performance.

Personal tutor: Each student will usually have a personal tutor allocated for the duration of the course. This allocation allows students the opportunity gain personal, professional and pastoral support in addition to the academic support on offer.

Practice-based mentor: When allocated to a practice placement, you are allocated a mentor who is usually a registered nurse who is responsible for your learning experiences and assessments during the period of allocation. Mentors are key members of the practice team and as such will have a busy workload. Therefore it is recommended that students follow the duty rota of their mentor as closely as possible to maximize learning opportunities.

University support networks: Universities offer comprehensive services for students. Publications summarizing these services are usually available and may be sent to students before a course starts. These services are user friendly and there to help and support you. The service include:

- Careers advice
- Chaplaincy and religious support
- Childcare information
- Counselling services
- Disability support
- Finance support, bursaries, fees, debt management
- Health surgeries
- Legal advice
- Library services
- Learning support
- Students union, for advice and recreational activities.

This support network also ensures that students have a framework for:

- gaining details of their academic and practice-related progress
- knowing the university regulations, e.g. relating to assessments, examinations, plagiarism, complaints procedures and behaviour
- knowing the university policies, e.g. relating to health and safety, fire and evacuation, dyslexia

- procedures for monitoring attendance, illness and absence
- professional requirements
- policy requirements, e.g. uniform, drug and health and safety policies relevant to practice experiences.

The student portfolio

Every student is required to maintain a professional portfolio. At the beginning of the course, you will be given a portfolio and guidelines for its completion during the course. This is yours to maintain and complete. Your lecturers and personal tutor will be particularly supportive regarding its completion. The portfolio is a collection of evidence relating to:

- your biographical details
- your previous educational experiences and qualifications
- action plans relating to key aspects of the course
- your course experiences and achievements
- summaries of key learning experiences during the course
- your reflections about what you have learned, how your competencies are developing, how you feel about your experiences and the learning that needs to take place.

It is a professional requirement for registered nurses to maintain a professional portfolio. Therefore the experience of maintaining a portfolio during the course is relevant to this. In the early stages as a registered nurse, some of the evidence contained in it from your course will be relevant and may support your professional development, e.g. job applications (see also Chapter 9). Additional sources of support are explored in detail in Chapter 8.

PROFESSIONAL ISSUES: PREPARING TO GAIN YOUR LICENCE TO PRACTISE NURSING

During a course, student nurses are expected to achieve a range of professional outcomes as you prepare to gain your licence to practise as a qualified nurse (see also Chapter 2). The NMC (2004a) has set out the competencies necessary for students undertaking pre-registration nursing courses (see Appendix 1). It offers guiding principles for the standard of pre-registration courses and states that for:

> ### Practice-centred learning
> The primary aim of pre-registration nursing programmes is to ensure that students are prepared to practise safely and effectively to such an extent that the protection of the public is assured. On this basis, it is a fundamental principle that programmes of preparation are practice-centred and directed towards the achievement of professional competence.
>
> (NMC, 2004a, p. 13)

In addition, the NMC (2004a) offers guidance relating to:

- Theory and practice integration
- Evidence-based practice and learning
- Responsibility: fitness for professional standing
- Adherence to the NMC Code of Professional Conduct: standards for conduct, performance and ethics
- Responsibility and accountability
- Ethical and legal obligations
- Respect for individuals and communities.

The NMC Code of Professional Conduct (NMC, 2004b; see Appendix 2) underpins the competencies and is an essential feature at all stages of pre-registration courses. It is essential for a student nurse to have an understanding of the NMC Code of Professional Conduct and the course requirements and competencies (see Appendix 1). These are explained and used to determine all aspects of the courses and are regularly referred to in teaching sessions and during practice placements, as well as being used to determine aspects of assessment and achievement (see also Chapter 2). Student nurses are expected to 'work within your level of understanding and competence and always under the direct supervision of a registered nurse or midwife' (NMC, 2002). In addition, student nurses must:

- respect the wishes of patients
- always accurately introduce themselves to patients as a student
- accept appropriate responsibilities

- safeguard patient confidentiality
- understand procedures for dealing with patient complaints (from NMC, 2002; see Appendix 3).

In *The NMC Code of Professional Conduct: standards for conduct, performance and ethics* (2004b; see Appendix 2), the NMC states that 'As a registered nurse, midwife or specialist community public health nurse, you are personally accountable for your practice. In caring for patients and clients, you must:

- respect the patient or client as an individual
- obtain consent before you give any treatment or care
- protect confidential information
- co-operate with others in the team
- maintain your professional knowledge and competence
- be trustworthy
- act to identify and minimize risk to patients and clients.'

Reflective activity

Compare the quote above from the NMC Code of Professional Conduct with the NMC Guide for Student Nurses (Appendix 3). Consider the way that you as a student are expected to comply with key professional standards while at the same time ensuring that you have appropriate supervision and support.

This process is all part of the preparation and education you receive during your course. As a student nurse, you are expected to act in a way that is appropriate to being in contact with the public, this is how you learn to become a safe and competent practitioner.

Summary

- Students can expect comprehensive teaching and support and feedback during their course.
- Students are expected to adhere to professional principles as part of their learning experience during the course.

YOUR NURSING COURSE

There are common features of nursing courses that are determined, as described, by legal and professional requirements. For 3-year courses, the structure of the course consists of the Common Foundation Programme which is 1 year in length, followed by the 2-year branch programme. This is organized over a 3-semester year. The 4-year courses tend to have a shorter academic year.

All students have to complete a total of 4600 hours of study and practice: 2300 theory and 2300 practice, as well as successfully completing the required course work and practice-based objectives and assessments to achieve the competencies.

Common Foundation Programme

The Common Foundation Programme (CFP) provides students with opportunities to gain a broad introduction to all aspects of nursing before entering their chosen branch. Therefore you will share most of this time with all the other students on the course, gaining experience in your chosen branch as well as the other branches of nursing. Increasingly, student nurses are taught alongside other students, e.g. physiotherapy, occupational health and medical students. Sharing experiences relating to a chosen profession is regarded as an important part of a health professional's education as well as learning about key topics together. There will be a mix of theoretical and practical input in most modules and you will be introduced to subjects such as:

- Nursing theory and practice
- Health and social policy
- Health promotion
- Health and safety policy and practice
- Primary health care
- Anatomy and physiology
- Communication studies
- Sociology applied to nursing
- Psychology applied to nursing
- Pharmacology
- Research appreciation
- Professional development
- Information technology and health care.

In addition, study skills, support with essay-writing techniques, time management and ensuring understanding of the available learning resources (e.g. the library) are included. You will be encouraged to develop your academic and learning skills. Effective decision-making and problem-solving abilities are essential skills for registered nurses so these are evaluated and assessed as part of the learning experiences during the whole course. Information technology has transformed many aspects of health care, patient record systems and education. These are explored during the course. You are expected to use a personal computer to produce assignments and projects, and support is on offer to ensure students are competent with this. Students also have an opportunity to realize an introduction to and learning experiences specific to their chosen branch programme as well as some exposure to experiences relating to the other branches of nursing. This provides all students with the opportunity to appreciate key aspects of care, practice and associated theory relevant to the other branches – but this is only an introduction.

Learning a range of practice skills is an important part of the course and individual modules and includes:

- Key aspects of patient care, e.g. observation skills, assessing blood pressure and temperature
- Interpersonal skills, e.g. patient interviewing, listening skills
- Caring for an immobile patient
- Safe lifting and handling techniques
- Resuscitation techniques
- Aseptic technique
- Hand washing and universal precautions
- Drug calculations
- Report writing.

Some of these skills are introduced as practical sessions within the HEI, which usually have facilities and skills centres designed as wards for this purpose. This initial introduction is linked to theoretical sessions to ensure that students understand the application of the research and evidence associated with the skills to their application in practice. Further experience is then necessary in practice placements to gain competence and confidence, apply the skills in differing circumstances to adapt them to various patients and their needs. It is acknowledged that not all practical skills can be introduced within practical sessions but are facilitated by mentors during practice experiences and in accordance with the objectives for the stage of the course. Assessment of the skills is part of this process and a record of achievement is essential to the successful completion of a stage of the course and progression to the next.

Branch programmes

Following successful completion of the CFP, students progress to their chosen branch programme in year 2 of the course. Detailed learning commences to fulfil the necessary branch specific competencies (see Appendix 1). Student experience relates to a range of branch-specific modules with associated theory and practice allocations. This allows students to gain experience caring for those requiring nursing and health care in a range of settings (see Chapters 4–7 for branch-specific details).

As the course progresses, so do the demands for developments in academic work, competence and professional development. The theoretical component of the course facilitates detailed study of key aspects of nursing including care management, policies, legal and professional perspectives relevant to patients and clients. The onus is on the students to develop more responsibility for their learning by undertaking an organized study programme for reading to support the programme, meeting deadlines for submitting work, taking advantage of tutorial opportunities and thoroughly preparing for lectures, lessons, seminars and tutorials.

The practice-based aspects of learning will usually offer a range of placements including:

- community-based experiences in primary care trusts (PCTs) and health centres, with district nurses, health visitors, community psychiatric nurses
- in schools with school nurses, nurseries e.g. for children's branch students
- in private sector hospitals and care homes, and in those offering social services provision, e.g. for learning disability and mental health branch students

- specialist units, e.g. coronary care, burns units (for adult branch students), forensic units (for mental health branch students) and neonatal units (for children's branch students).

Elective placements are experiences that students have chosen under the guidance of course lecturers. These may be in the UK or aboard and complement the chosen branch, stage of the course, level of learning and interests of the student.

As the branch programme progresses into the final year of the course, so the work intensifies and realization that, on successful completion of the course, first posts as a registered nurse needs to be planned for. Successful completion of the branch programme and the course as a whole will allow you entry in the nurses part of the NMC register. The NMC register has three parts:

- Nurses
- Midwives
- Specialist Community Public Health Nurses.

And finally – career advice, support and preparation for the transition between being a student and becoming a registered nurse is a key focus. Making the all important career choices is explored in Chapter 9, but the influences for these first post choices will often relate to placements that have been part of the course and the positive relationships, experiences and feedback received from registered practitioners and course lecturers.

Whatever your decision and wherever your first post takes you, this marks the beginning of a valuable, worthwhile career. May you grow and benefit from it as well as find satisfaction from supporting those who are vulnerable and in varying states of health.

REFERENCES

Department of Health (2000) *The NHS Plan*. London: DoH.
Department of Health (2003) *Financial Help for Health Care Students*, 6th edn. London: DoH.
Department of Health (2004) *The NHS Improvement Plan: putting people at the heart of public services*. London: DoH.
Department of Health (2005) *The NHS Improvement Plan: putting people at the heart of public services: executive summary*. London: DoH.

Henderson V (1966) *The Nature of Nursing.* New York: Macmillan.

Nursing and Midwifery Council (2002) *An NMC Guide for Students of Nursing and Midwifery.* London: NMC.

Nursing and Midwifery Council (2004a) *Standards of Proficiency for Pre-registration Nursing Education.* London: NMC.

Nursing and Midwifery Council (2004b) *The NMC Code of Professional Conduct: standards for conduct, performance and ethics.* London: NMC.

Royal College of Nursing (2004) *The Future Nurse: the RCN vision.* London: RCN.

ANNOTATED FURTHER READING

Burnard P (2002) *Learning Human Skills. An experiential and reflective guide for nurses and health care professionals,* 4th edn. Oxford: Butterworth-Heinemann. This book supports two important themes for nurses: the development of effective nurse–patient relationships and learning through reflective practice.

Cronin P, Rawlings-Anderson K (2004) *Knowledge for Contemporary Nursing Practice.* London: Mosby. This book is a useful introduction to the relationship between nursing knowledge and nursing practice. Reference to key writers on nursing and key professional issues, e.g. how care is managed, is included.

Hinchliff S, Norman SE, Schober JE (eds) (2003) *Nursing Practice and Health Care,* 4th edn. London: Arnold. A popular and comprehensive text for all student nurses preparing for registration. It provides essential information in 19 chapters relating to a wide range of professional issues including patient care, professional development and care delivery as they relate to the NMC competency framework.

Lanoe N (2002) *Ogier's Reading Research,* 3rd edn. Edinburgh: Ballière Tindall. It is a professional requirement to apply up-to-date information and research to practice. This book is a valuable introduction to this and to the process of research appreciation.

Nursing and Midwifery Council (2004) *Guidelines for the Administration of Medicines.* London: NMC. The NMC produces a range of publications to support professional practice and professional development for registered nurses. This document contains guidelines relating to the administration of medicines.

Nursing and Midwifery Council (2005) *Guidelines for Records and Record Keeping.* London: NMC. As above, these guidelines support standards for record keeping.

Royal College of Nursing (2004) *The Future Nurse: the RCN vision.* London: RCN. A brief but valuable account of issues relating to nursing and the future role of nurses.

Whitehead E, Mason, T (2003) *Study Skills for Nurses.* London: Sage. This is one of a range of texts aimed at supporting the study necessary during a course and covers a number of important skills including time management, exam technique, producing assignments and reflective practice.

USEFUL WEBSITES

National library resources and key sources of information

NHS knowledge grid for health

England: www.library.nhs.uk
N Ireland: www.honni.qub.ac.uk
Scotland: www.elib.scot.nhs.uk
Wales: www.wales.nhs.uk

National Service Frameworks. National standards for care groups and services available at www.dh.gov.uk/PolicyAndGuidance/HealthAndSocialCareTopics – these include coronary heart disease, cancer, paediatric intensive care, mental health, older people, diabetes, long-term conditions, renal and children.

National Institute for Health and Clinical Excellence (NICE). www.nice.org.uk – guidance on arthritis, asthma, cancer, diabetes, infections and infectious diseases, lung cancer, nutritional disorders and violence.

Professional issues, Agenda for Change

For further general information

Department of Health. www.dh.gov.uk
NHS Modernisation Agency. www.modern.nhs.uk/agendafor change
Nursing Standard. www.nursing-standard.co.uk
RCN Agenda for Change. www.rcn.org.uk/agendaforchange
NHS Scotland. www.show.scot.nhs.uk/sehd/paymodernisation/AfC/index.htm
NHS Wales. www.wales.nhs.uk
The Northern Ireland Executive. www.nics.gov.uk/

2

Professional Issues and Implications for Practice

Carol Ash

INTRODUCTION

Individuals entering or considering application to a pre-registration nursing programme in higher education need to be aware that as well as embarking on a nursing career they are also preparing to become members of a profession. In practice, this means that one learns nursing within the framework and standards published by the regulatory body, the Nursing and Midwifery Council (NMC, 2004a).

The route to registration and the license to practise is clearly defined through the NMC (2004b) standards of proficiency for pre-registration nursing education including practice and conduct (see Appendix 1). The educational standards set by the NMC apply to pre-registration students at the entry point to an educational programme as the NMC is empowered to determine the entry level, type and length of the programme (NMC, 2004b).

The implications for students preparing for registration and the licence to practise are detailed in the publication *An NMC Guide for Students of Nursing and Midwifery* (NMC, 2002a; see Appendix 3). This leaflet gives brief guidelines for students on the role and functions of the NMC and also provides clear guidance on clinical experience for students. The overall aim of the NMC is to establish and improve standards of nursing care to protect the public. Therefore, nursing students should familiarize themselves with the guidelines for professional practice identified in *The NMC Code of Professional Conduct: standards for conduct, performance and ethics* (see Appendix 2). The code of professional conduct handbook (NMC, 2004a) has been included in Appendix 2 but it can also be obtained from the university providing the educational programme or from the NMC website.

Nurses must respond to the changing health care needs of the patients and communities they serve (NMC, 2004b). Therefore, education for nursing practice must be designed to meet the needs of health services as well as the specific needs of the profession. The demands of professional practice are increasingly complex in terms of the rapidly changing nature of health care provision and the expectations of patients and communities. The aim of this chapter is to explore the professional background to nursing and the implications for students preparing for a nursing career. The key areas that will be explored in this chapter include:

- Nursing as a profession
- The framework for professional practice
- Professional self-regulation and accountability for practice
- The role of professional organizations and trade unions
- Dilemmas and conflicts in practice.

NURSING AS A PROFESSION

Traditionally a profession has been characterized by the provision of a unique service to society requiring specialized knowledge and skills, and the control of education and standards of practice through a statutory body. Additionally, a profession usually protects the public interest through a code of professional conduct based on ethical and legal principles (Davies, 1995). Examples include the professions of medicine and dentistry. These are acknowledged as professions because education and preparation of practitioners has been characterized by a lengthy full time university education as well as the development of clinical competence within clinical practice settings. Professional practice is underpinned by research and the evidence is used to support practice. Many practitioners participate in the research process, therefore increasing the knowledge base in their particular area of practice. These recognized professions are also self-regulating and have developed and maintained professional autonomy.

The principle whether nursing can be defined as a profession continues to be debated by students and registered nurses. Twenty years ago, Jane Salvage questioned whether nursing should want to be a profession and challenged nurses to define the term profession (Salvage, 1985). Nursing has struggled in the past to develop a body of knowledge that is uniquely nursing knowledge. However, the advent of funded nursing research and the development of university-based education for students and registered nurses has assisted nursing in the quest for professional recognition.

It may be helpful here to distinguish between professional conduct commonly referred to as professionalism and professionalization. The latter term is generally understood to be the route that an occupational group takes to establish the rules, standards and procedures of a profession (Davies, 1995).

The central role of nursing is to care for patients and the professional and caring side of professional practice is at the core of nursing. Professionalism needs to be informed by models of caring. New professionalism promotes partnerships with patients and the empowerment of patients as being more important than the role of the expert (Davies, 1995). Partnerships with patients are based on this premise and care management is a joint endeavour between patient and nurse. This principle underpins modern nursing with the registered nurse acknowledging personal and professional accountability for practice.

Registered nurses act as role models for students as well as mentors and assessors of practice. Davies

(1995) argues that students of nursing learn to act in a professional way in their everyday work with patients and colleagues. However, students must learn to practise nursing in accordance with the NMC code of professional conduct (NMC, 2004a) within an ethical and legal framework that ensures patient interest and well-being.

Summary

- Professions require specialized knowledge and skills.
- Education and standards of practice are regulated by a statutory body.
- A code of professional conduct based on legal and ethical principles determines professional behaviour (Davies, 1995, p. 133).

Development of nursing as a profession

The history of nursing has been well documented (Baly, 1997). Students may gain insights and enhance their understanding of the influences on the developments in nursing by reading some of the suggested texts listed at the end of the chapter. Key landmarks (Box 2.1) will be identified in this part of the chapter in terms of the progression towards professional registration and self-regulation.

Box 2.1 Key landmarks influencing the development of nursing as a profession

- Nurse Registration Act 1919
- Nurses, Midwives and Health Visitors Act 1979, amended in 1992
- The United Kingdom Central Council for Nursing, Midwifery and Health Visiting code of professional conduct (1984)
- The United Kingdom Council for Nursing, Midwifery and Health Visiting Commission for Nursing, and Midwifery Education (1999)
- The Nursing and Midwifery Council (2002)

The Nurse Registration Act 1919

A register for nurses was established before 1889 for women who had undertaken a year's training. Subsequent campaigns by prominent nurse leaders and medical practitioners of the time resulted in The Nurse Registration Acts of 1919 and the first principles of nurse registration and regulation emerged as a result of these Acts of Parliament.

Subsequently, the formation of the general nursing councils gave responsibility to the councils for professional discipline and regulation. Standards of training were established for nurses to register as qualified practitioners (Glover, 1999). This was an important landmark for nursing as the framework for professional self-regulation was established as well as the acceptability of nursing as a reasonable career.

United Kingdom Central Council for Nursing, Midwifery and Health Visiting

The general nursing councils existed for over 50 years until the Nurses, Midwives and Health Visitors Act of 1979 resulted in the establishment of the United Kingdom Central Council (UKCC) for Nursing, Midwifery and Health Visiting and the four national boards for England, Wales, Northern Ireland and Scotland. The UKCC was established in 1983, although it had existed in shadow form since 1981. This regulatory body replaced nine other statutory training bodies which had existed by Acts of Parliament or ministerial decisions whose powers had been fragmented across professions and the UK. The new statutory body, was now responsible for maintaining the register for nurses, midwives and health visitors (Pyne, 1995).

The UKCC recognized that its main responsibility was to protect the public through standards of education, training and professional conduct. The Nurses, Midwives and Health Visitors Act 1979 clearly stated that the principal function of the council was to establish and improve standards of training and professional conduct for registered nurses, registered midwives and registered health visitors. A statutory instrument (Rule 18a) formalizing the level at which a registered nurse could perform and personal accountability for practice was acknowledged.

Development of self-regulation and professional accountability

The first code of professional conduct was implemented in 1984 and the principle of professional accountability of registered nurses was established (Dimond, 1995). The guiding principle was that upon registration and following education and training, patients could reasonably expect a nurse to be competent and to be able to practise safely. Additionally, registered nurses had a duty of care to their patients by the very nature of the nurse–patient relationship (Glover, 1999). The duty of care principle and implications for registered nurses and students will be discussed in more detail later in this chapter.

The Nurse, Midwives and Health Visitors Act was amended in 1992. The amended Act reinforced the principles of professional self-regulation to be exercised in the public interest. Changes to the constitution were made which allowed for two-thirds of the membership of the council to be democratically elected by the professions and one-third to be appointed by the Secretary of State. Rule 18 of the Nurses, Midwives and Health Visitors Amendment Act (1992) determined that practice should be underpinned by identified competencies.

A number of separate criminal cases, involving doctors and nurses in the early 1990s attracted media attention and public interest. The government subsequently commissioned an independent review of professional regulation and the report was published in 1998 (JM Consulting, 1998). The perception at that time was that there was a need to make professional self-regulation more responsive, open and accountable in terms of public confidence. The report provided the basis for the most recent reforms in professional regulation and resulted in the demise of the UKCC and the establishment of the NMC in 2002.

The Commission for Nursing and Midwifery Education

Nursing and Midwifery Education was integrated into higher education in the early 1990s, and a new curriculum, Project 2000, was implemented. Nursing students were able to access the resources of higher education institutions (HEIs) in pursuit of an academic and professional qualification.

A subsequent evaluation of Project 2000 raised some concerns among employers and the public in terms of a nurse's fitness to practise at the point of registration. As a result, the UKCC Commission for Nursing and Midwifery Education were asked 'to prepare a way forward for pre-registration nursing and midwifery education that enables fitness for practice based on health care need' (UKCC Commission for Nursing and Midwifery Education, 1999, p. 2).

The commission recognized that the basic principles of Project 2000 were sound in terms of the preparation of practitioners to participate in the planning, assessment and development of services. However, the perception of employers and to some extent the public, was that newly qualified nurses did not possess the practice skills expected of them. This situation improved when registrants gained experience after a short time in work (UKCC, 1999).

Employers concerns were addressed through a re-focusing of pre-registration programmes on outcomes-based competency principles which have subsequently been developed by HIEs in close collaboration with service providers. The effective delivery of integration of theory and practice within the educational programme was considered to be vital to produce 'knowledgeable doers' (UKCC, 1999).

Increased flexibility in terms of access by students from differing personal, academic and vocational backgrounds to educational programmes was recommended. In addition, closer working partnerships between HIEs and service providers was considered to be important in support of teaching and learning in practice (UKCC, 1999).

Establishment of the Nursing and Midwifery Council

A smaller council and a streamlined regulatory framework for nurses, midwives and health visitors was established following an interim council that managed the change for a two-year period. The four national boards were disbanded and the current Nursing and Midwifery Council became operational in April 2002. The NMC is required by the Nursing and Midwifery Order (2001) to establish and maintain a register of qualified nurses and midwives and to establish standards of proficiency

required by entrants to the different parts of the register to ensure safe and effective practice. The NMC also has additional powers to deal with professional misconduct and individual health issues, and employers and the public are able to establish the status of nurse registrants.

The professional register was simplified in 2004. There are now three parts to the register for nurses, midwives and specialist community public health nurses. Additionally, new registrants will be identified in terms of the branch in which the standards of proficiency have been met (NMC, 2004a). Details of the structure and functions of the NMC can be found in Appendix 2.

Summary

- Nurse Registration Act 1919 established the first principles of nurse registration; standards of training identified.
- Nurses, Midwives and Health Visitors Act 1979, amended 1992.
- First code of professional conduct for Nurses, Midwives and Health Visitors in 1984.
- Nursing and Midwifery Council established in 2002.

FRAMEWORK FOR PROFESSIONAL PRACTICE

Nursing is a profession grounded in practice, therefore, professional competence is mandatory in terms of fitness to practise as a registered nurse. The NMC publication (NMC, 2004b), defines the standards of proficiency for pre-registration education and links fitness for practice to fitness for purpose, professional academic awards and professional standing.

Fitness for practice is generally understood to mean the achievement of the required standards of proficiency (previously competencies) in preparation for entry to the professional register. Fitness for purpose is linked to the ability of registered nurses to respond to the changing needs of the health service and the communities that they serve (NMC, 2004b). In practice, registered nurses should be able to function competently in clinical practice, and accept responsibility for their professional development.

The NMC provides a confidential professional advice service for registered nurses and midwives as well as other health care workers and the public. Advice is focused on the NMC's standards and guidelines for practice, education and conduct (NMC, 2002b).

Standards of education and proficiency

Educational programmes are based on the principle that nursing is practice based with patient/clients at the centre of care. Guiding principles (Box 2.2) relate to the professional standards of proficiency and fitness to practise. The standards of proficiency must be reflected in all programmes of preparation for the register, and students must achieve the standards of proficiency in a specific branch of nursing before they can apply for registration. Formerly, the standards of educational and practice outcomes were known as competencies (NMC, 2002b). The competencies have now been adopted as standards of proficiency (NMC, 2004b).

Box 2.2 Guiding principles for nurse education (NMC, 2004b, p. 23)

- Evidence should inform practice
- Students are actively involved in nursing care delivery under supervision
- The NMC Code of Professional Conduct: standards for conduct, performance and ethics, applies to all practice interventions
- Skills and knowledge are transferable
- Research underpins practice
- The importance of life-long learning and continuing professional development is recognized

---

The standards of proficiency are underpinned by standards of education with four related domains (Box 2.3). The domains may apply to more than one standard of proficiency. The standards of proficiency are incremental in terms of entry to the branch programmes and subsequent completion of the educational programme. It is essential that

students develop the knowledge and skills underpinning clinical practice in combination with an understanding of the professional role. Nursing care is delivered within a professional practice framework consistent with the values of the professional group (Fryer, 2003).

Box 2.3 The four domains

- Professional and ethical practice
- Care delivery
- Care management
- Personal and professional development

Source: NMC, 2004b, pp. 26–34

The implications for nursing students are that they learn nursing within this framework and are novice members of the group. The NMC (2004b) code of professional conduct provides the framework for registered nurses in terms of standards, conduct and performance, therefore, students should use the code as a key reference point. The primary aim of the NMC and the profession is to ensure that students practise nursing safely and effectively ensuring that the public is protected.

Continuing professional development

An essential feature of professional practice is the need for continuing professional development. Registered nurses must accept responsibility for their continuing education and life-long learning. They are now required to demonstrate responsibility for their own learning through the development of a portfolio of learning and practice and recognition of when further learning and development may be required (NMC, 2002c). The maintenance of professional knowledge and competence is not an

---

Reflective activity

Identify the following: (i) the key principles in terms of the license to practise nursing (ii) the four professional domains where students need to achieve standards of proficiency and (iii) the key responsibilities of the registered nurse in the continuation of fitness for practice.

option for registered nurses. This requirement is stated in the code of professional conduct (NMC, 2004a) and is a condition for continuing registration and the licence to practise (see Chapter 9).

Current developments in the NHS

Current developments in the National Health Service (NHS) include the establishment of the NHS Modernisation Agency supporting the current modernization of the NHS as the major provider of health care in the UK. The present government agenda is to improve and monitor the patient experience at different levels of care. Examples include the reduction of patient waiting times for surgery and in out-patient departments. The establishment of foundation hospitals is a government initiative designed to give flagship hospitals more autonomy and financial control.

The NHS Plan (Department of Health (DoH), 2000) and *The NHS Plan – an action guide for nurses, midwives and health visitors* (DoH, 2001) are strategic plans aimed at the provision of a health service focused on the needs of patients. A series of documents aimed at different professional groups within the NHS identifies organizational and professional needs to be addressed to improve services and to provide opportunities for staff. Similarly, 'Agenda for Change' determines new frameworks for the employment of nurses within the NHS in terms of pay and employment conditions. 'Agenda for Change' (DoH, 2004) recognizes the contribution of nurses as key players in the delivery of effective health care.

Modern nursing is now supported by a philosophy and practice focused on the promotion of standards of nursing care and the quality of service offered to patients and clients. Therefore, collaboration with other agencies, for example, NHS trusts, voluntary organizations and other health care professionals is vital if students are to learn nursing to the required standards of proficiency and to work within multi-disciplinary teams (see example in Box 2.4). Students will also need to understand the clinical and professional roles of other health workers and to respect and use the knowledge and skills necessary for effective patient care.

The complex and rapidly changing health care environment needs to be informed by evidence to

---

> ## Box 2.4 The multi-disciplinary team
>
> - Nurses: specialist community public health nurses and midwives
> - Doctors
> - Physiotherapists
> - Radiographers
> - Pharmacists
> - Occupational therapists
> - Technicians
> - Significant others

support practice (NMC, 2004b). This principle requires students and registered nurses to search for the best available evidence, using research outcomes and evidence emerging from practice.

Summary

- Students learn nursing supported by an academic programme provided by an HEI in combination with learning in practice.
- Students must complete the educational programme and achieve the NMC (2004b) standards of proficiency before they are eligible to be considered for registration on the professional register.
- Students learn nursing within a professional framework that is determined by the regulatory body, the Nursing and Midwifery Council (NMC, 2004a).

PROFESSIONAL SELF-REGULATION AND ACCOUNTABILITY FOR PRACTICE

The core function of the regulatory body, the NMC, is to establish and improve the standards of nursing, midwifery and health visiting to protect the public. Its key tasks include (NMC, 2002a):

- maintaining a register for all nurses, midwives and health visitors
- setting standards and guidelines for nursing, midwifery and health visiting education, practice and conduct
- providing advice on professional standards for registrants

- providing quality assurance for nursing and midwifery education
- consideration of allegations of misconduct or unfitness to practise due to ill health.

The powers of the NMC are detailed in the Nursing and Midwifery Order 2001 and are available to students on the NMC website (www.nmc-uk.org).

The NMC Code of Professional Conduct

The NMC Code of Professional Conduct: standards for conduct, performance and ethics sets the standards for practice and defines the responsibilities of accountable registered nurses (NMC, 2004a). The code is clear that registered nurses should act at all times in a manner to safeguard and promote the interests of individual patients and clients and to enhance the reputation of the profession. The code provides a framework for professional decision-making, therefore, professional behaviour is governed by explicit standards. The purpose of The NMC Code of Professional Conduct: standards for conduct, performance and ethics (p. 4) is to:

- inform the professions of the standard of professional conduct required of them in the exercise of their professional accountability
- inform the public, other professions and employers of the standard of professional conduct they can expect of a registered practitioner.

Accountability has been defined as 'the requirement that each nurse is answerable and responsible for the outcome of his or her professional actions' (Pennels, 1997). The NMC states that registered nurses, midwives and specialist community public health nurses are personally accountable for their practice and answerable for their actions and omissions regardless of advice or directions from other health care professionals (NMC, 2004a). Nurses are also accountable to (Dimond, 1995):

- the patient – through a duty of care, and the common law of negligence and through civil law
- the public – through criminal law
- the profession – through The NMC Code of Professional Conduct: standards for conduct, performance and ethics
- the employer – through contract law.

Duty of care

The duty of care principle has been established for many years. Nurses have a duty of care to their patients when there is a pre-existing relationship between nurse and patient and the patient has presented for potential treatment or care or has accepted treatment or care. The duty of care is underpinned by the concept of 'reasonableness' which is the standard defined by the law (Glover, 1999). The NMC (2004a) defines the concept of 'reasonable' by citing the case of Bolam v Friern Barnet Hospital Management Committee (1957):

> The test is the standard of the ordinary skilled man exercising and professing to have that special skill. A man need not possess the highest expert skill at the risk of being found negligent. … it is sufficient if he exercises the skill of an ordinary man exercising that particular art.

This definition is referred to as the Bolam Test and arose out of case law and applies to all health professionals including nurses. The registered nurse has discharged the duty of care if the actions carried out are reasonable. However, the duty of care may be breached through an act or omission that is usually foreseeable in terms of causing injury to the patient (Dimond, 1995).

This definition has established the principle of personal and professional accountability for registered nurses in practice, and has been used in legal cases involving alleged professional negligence. However, if registered nurses practise within the terms of their employment and guidelines defined by their employers, vicarious liability on the part of the employer may apply if a patient pursues a civil claim against a nurse. This means that the employer will take legal responsibility for the registered nurse's actions if the actions took place during their employment. The NMC (2004a) advises registered nurses to establish their insurance status and if their employers do not accept vicarious liability then the regulatory body recommends that registrants obtain professional indemnity insurance.

Implications for nursing students

Pre-registration students are not professionally accountable because they are not qualified or eligible to register with the NMC. Therefore, nursing students cannot be professionally accountable for their actions or omissions by the NMC. The registered nurse supervising the learning activities of a student is professionally responsible for the actions or omissions of students (NMC, 2002a). However, students are personally accountable for their actions or omissions and can be held to account by the university providing the educational programme, or by the law (NMC, 2002a).

It is essential that nursing students understand that they should learn nursing practice through the direct supervision of a registered nurse. Although students are not professionally accountable they are responsible for their actions. Registered nurses are accountable for delegated activities but the NMC guidance for students states clearly that they should only work within their level of understanding and competence and always under the direct supervision of a registered nurse (NMC, 2002a). Students should also acknowledge that patients have the right to refuse to allow students to participate in their caring and the rights of patients have priority over the students' rights to knowledge and experience (NMC, 2002a).

Reflective activity

Define the personal and professional accountability of the registered nurse and the personal accountability of students for their practice.

Discuss the rights of patients, and the legal duty of care to patients, the public, employers and the profession.

ROLE OF PROFESSIONAL ORGANIZATIONS AND TRADE UNIONS

Professional organizations and trade unions play a vital role in the support of nurses in terms of employment conditions, including pay and working conditions as well as improved education. They are also instrumental in terms of influencing decision-making and represent nurses at the highest levels of management and policy making (Salvage, 2003).

The Royal College of Nursing

The Royal College of Nursing (RCN) was founded in 1916 and is an accredited independent professional union, working with political parties in the interests of patients and nurses. On its website the RCN states that it is 'the leading professional union for nursing' and campaigns on behalf of the profession, influencing the development of nursing practice. The RCN is also active in lobbying the government in safeguarding the interests of patients to ensure that the views of the profession are heard (RCN, 2005).

The college is managed by nurses and works locally and internationally to promote nursing as a profession as well as the interests of individual nurses. The objectives of the Royal Charter are detailed on the RCN website (www.rcn.org.uk). The RCN offers a wide range of services for registered nurses and students (Box 2.5).

Box 2.5 RCN services

- Advice on work-related problems
- Legal representation
- Education and professional development activities
- Professional advice
- Counselling and personal advice service
- Immigration advice
- Support and activities for nursing students
- Free publications on nursing
- Health care and employment issues (largest library in Europe)

The RCN legal services offer an indemnity service that provides cover for students as well as other RCN members. Details of the scheme can be found on the website. The conditions for students are that they only undertake responsibilities that they have trained for and feel competent to perform under supervision. This is an important point and students should refer to the NMC (2002a) guide for students of nursing and midwifery (see Appendix 3). All student members of the RCN are automatically members of the RCN Association of Nursing Students and have access to RCN-trained stewards representing students and staff on the campuses of most HEIs.

Other trade unions and organizations

UNISON is one of the larger trade unions and members work in the NHS, colleges and schools, the police force and other public sector services. It differs from the RCN as the membership is open to all public sector workers, with health care membership comprising one of six employment groups.

Unions address issues such as discrimination in the work place and negotiate agreements that improve the working lives of members. UNISON benefits include representation for members, legal services, education and training advice, as well as help with pay and conditions of service. Additionally, UNISON offers health and safety advice and is also known for campaigning and lobbying on key issues affecting members and the public. It is also the largest union affiliated to the Trades Union Congress (TUC).

The TUC claims that 'it campaigns for a fair deal at work and for social justice at home and abroad' (see www. tuc.org.uk). Students may obtain further information from the TUC website and the websites of the organizations listed there.

Other professional associations and organizations have been established representing the interests of nurses working in clinical and non-clinical specialities. Examples include associations representing theatre nurses, critical care nurses, and nurses working in accident and emergency departments. Similarly, specialist community public health nurses have their own organization. The RCN has also established research, education and practice forums for the exchange of ideas and the promotion of

---

Reflective activity

Define the role of professional organizations and trade unions influencing the development of the NHS. What are the advantages/disadvantages of belonging to a professional organization or trade union?

What is professional indemnity and when is it necessary?

---

developments in practice. Representatives of the RCN and other unions visit higher education sites to communicate the benefits of joining their unions. Students need to gain information in terms of membership benefits and costs and avail themselves of the opportunity to discuss these details with the union representatives.

DILEMMAS AND CONFLICTS IN PRACTICE

Members of the public and patients do not always understand the distinction between registered nurses, student nurses, and other health care personnel working in health care environments. The NMC recently reported that it had received enquiries relating to the use of the title of 'nurse' (NMC, 2005). The title of nurse is not prohibited by law, however, the title of 'registered nurse' is protected by the Nursing and Midwifery Act 1983 and it is a criminal offence to falsely and deliberately present as a registered nurse or midwife. The NMC suggests that the title of nurse has major implications for patients, employees and employers as patients have the right to expect and demand the level of education, skills and knowledge from any person who uses this title.

The dilemma for student nurses is that patients and relatives may be unaware of their student status and seek information and professional advice inappropriately. This is particularly important when patients and relatives are distressed and are unhappy about treatment or care or when a complaint is being made. Nursing students are advised by the NMC (2002a) to introduce themselves accurately to patients directly or on the telephone and to make it clear to patients and the public that they are pre-registration students and not registered practitioners. The advice of a registered nurse, preferably the supervising nurse, should be sought if patients are unhappy about their treatment or care.

Students should be aware of local complaints procedures. Shortages of qualified nursing staff and the resulting pressures of an excessive workload may place additional pressures on student nurses. Students are advised by the NMC (2002a) not to participate in any procedure for which they have not been fully prepared or have been adequately supervised. Students should discuss issues with their supervising nurse as soon as possible and with the link lecturer from the HEI. It is important to communicate concerns in terms of patient safety and it is vital that students should be advised to exercise caution if they are unsure of their proficiency in particular situations.

Students should also familiarize themselves with the local policies for the handling and storage of records (NMC, 2002a). Entries to patient records by students should be counter-signed by a registered nurse. In addition, students should not refer to confidential information in their written assignments that could identify patients. Students must work within the framework of the code of professional practice (NMC, 2004a) and protect confidential information.

The nature and extent of supervision of students by registered nurses in practice areas has caused some concerns to students mainly due to the shift patterns of supervising nurses as well as staff sickness and annual leave. However, students should discuss supervision issues with their practice supervisors and link lecturers at the HIE as well as nurse managers when appropriate.

It is in the best interests of students on entry to the educational programme to read the student regulations and familiarize themselves with the curriculum as well as the guidelines for the attainment of the academic award. Guidelines are available in terms of the criteria for the presentation and completion of written assessments and the achievement of practice outcomes, as well as the resources available to students for academic support. The RCN Association of Nursing Students has detailed information on its website in terms of issues of interest to nursing students. Other support mechanisms for students are also detailed in Chapter 8 of this book.

Student nurses come from different age groups, and educational and cultural backgrounds. This diversity adds a wealth of human experience to a student nurse's educational experience as well as future nursing practice. Many students have external responsibilities such as part-time employment and the need to care for other family members. Personal conflict may occur between the effort required to achieve the required standards of proficiency in practice and the attainment of the

academic award, as well as managing responsibilities external to the university. Additionally, students are encouraged to participate in the social side of university life. The management of these priorities is an issue that students need to reflect on and address in terms of allocating dedicated time for study.

Students learning nursing are also learning to become professional practitioners within a complex health care environment. Many students respond to these challenges positively and are able to look forward with optimism to an interesting and fulfilling career in nursing. Nursing offers an exciting variety of career opportunities and further details are explored in Chapter 9.

Summary

- Students should practise nursing within the standards identified by *The NMC Code of Professional Conduct: standards for conduct, performance and ethics.*
- Students should not participate in any procedure when they are not fully prepared or have not been supervised.
- Students should discuss problems in practice with their nurse supervisor and personal tutor.
- In written assignments students should not refer to confidential information that could identify patients.
- Students need to prioritize responsibilities and allocate time for continuing study.

GLOSSARY

In the context of this chapter the meanings of the following words are described:

Accountable	Responsible for something or someone
Competent	Possessing the skills and abilities required for lawful, safe and effective professional practice without direct supervision
Evidence-based practice	Analysing, critiquing and using research and other forms of evidence for practice
Patient/client	Any individual or group using a health service
Practice-centred learning	Programmes of preparation are directed towards the achievement of proficiency

| Standards of proficiency | Standards to be met by applicants to different parts of the professional register. Standards necessary for safe and effective practice. Previously referred to as competencies |
| Theory and practice integration | Theoretical knowledge that underpins practice |

REFERENCES

Baly M (1997) *Florence Nightingale and the Nursing Legacy.* London: Whurr Publishers.

Bolam *v* Friern Barnet Hospital Management Committee (1957) In: *The NMC Code of Professional Conduct: standards for conduct, performance and ethics.* London: NMC (p. 5).

Davies C (1995) *Gender and the Professional Predicament in Nursing.* Buckingham: Open University Press.

Dimond B (1995) *Legal Aspects of Nursing.* London: Prentice Hall.

Department of Health (2000) *The NHS Plan.* London: DoH.

Department of Health (2001) *The NHS Plan – an action guide for nurses, midwives and health visitors.* London: DoH.

Department of Health (2004) *Agenda for Change: final agreement.* London: DoH.

Fryer N (2003) Principles of Professional Practice. In: Hinchcliff S, Norman SE, Schober JE (eds), *Nursing Practice and Healthcare*, 4th edn. London: Hodder Arnold.

Glover D (1999) Accountability. *Nursing Times Monographs.* No.27.

JM Consulting (1998) *The Regulation of Nurses, Midwives and Health Visitors.* Bristol: JM Consulting Ltd.

Nurses, Midwives and Health Visitors Act (1979) London: HMSO.

Nurses, Midwives and Health Visitors Amendment Act (1992) London: HMSO.

Nursing and Midwifery Order (2001), Norwich, The Stationery Office (www.opsi.gov.uk).

Nursing and Midwifery Council (2002a) *An NMC Guide for Students of Nursing and Midwifery.* London: NMC.

Nursing and Midwifery Council (2002b) *Professional Advice from the NMC.* London: NMC.

Nursing and Midwifery Council (2002c) *Supporting Nurses and Midwives Through Lifelong Learning.* London: NMC.

Nursing and Midwifery Council (2004a) *The NMC Code of Professional Conduct: standards for conduct, performance and ethics.* London: NMC.

Nursing and Midwifery Council (2004b) *Standards of Proficiency for Pre-registration Nursing Education.* London: NMC

Nursing and Midwifery Council (2005) Using nurse as a title. *NMC News* (10) 9.

Pennels C (1997) Nursing and the Law: clinical responsibility. *Professional Nurse* 13(3): 162–164.

Pennels C (1998) *Nursing and the Law.* London: Professional Nurse E/Map Healthcare.

Pyne R (1995) The professional dimension. In: Tingle J, Cribb A (eds), *Nursing Law and Ethics.* Oxford: Blackwell Science, pp. 36–58.

Royal College of Nursing (2005) *Agenda for Change – a guide to the pay, terms and conditions in the NHS.* London: RCN.

Salvage J (1985) *The Politics of Nursing.* London: Heinemann.

Salvage J (2003) Nursing today and tomorrow. In Hinchcliff S, Norman SE, Schober JE (eds), *Nursing Practice and Health Care*, 4th edn. London: Hodder Arnold.

United Kingdom Central Council (1999) *Fitness for Practice.* The UKCC Commission for Nursing and Midwifery Education. London: UKCC.

ANNOTATED FURTHER READING

Hinchliff S, Norman SE, Schober JE (eds) (2003) *Nursing Practice and Health Care*, 4th edn. London: Arnold. A comprehensive textbook suitable for pre-registration students as well as registered nurses. A wide range of professional and practice issues provide the reader with essential information including issues for reflection and debate. This edited book has contributions from nurses working in practice and nurses teaching and researching in HEIs.

Tingle J, Cribb A (eds) (1995) *Nursing Law and Ethics.* Oxford: Blackwell Science. A useful edited book for pre-registration students analysing the legal and ethical background to modern day health care from a historical perspective. Students may use this book for reference in terms of background information leading to the current legislation and professional regulation.

USEFUL WEBSITES

Department of Health. www.doh.gov.uk
Nursing and Midwifery Council. www.nmc-uk.org
Royal College of Nursing. www.rcn.org.uk
UNISON. www.unison.org.uk

3

Recent Developments in Nursing Practice

Veronica Bishop

INTRODUCTION

The aim of this chapter is to introduce the reader to recent developments in nursing practice, and how they have influenced nursing and health care. Constant changes in politics and ever-increasing advances in technology have combined to present greater challenges than ever in meeting the health demands of the UK population. Therefore the need for practitioners to develop support mechanisms will be stressed. Nursing has a complex history and key landmarks are summarized in Table 3.1. These serve to complement the three main sections of this chapter, which are as follows:

- Developments in clinical practice
- Research and development in nursing
- Support for clinical excellence

DEVELOPMENTS IN CLINICAL PRACTICE: THE LYNCHPIN OF PROFESSIONAL NURSING

This section stresses the importance of clinical practice to nursing, not only with a view to improving patient services, but also in terms of political power and the associated ability to shape the future of the nursing profession rather than it being shaped by others. Examples of clinical innovations will be discussed, such as clinical supervision, clinical governance and evidence-based practice. Relevant publications will be identified to assist the student to grasp a foothold in the political and clinical environment which makes up the National Health Service (NHS). Key reports include the United Kingdom Central Council (UKCC) 1999 report *Fitness for Practice* with its stress on clinical support, and its recognition of the need for collaboration between the NHS and higher education.

Clinical practice is fundamental to nursing. The power and value of nursing is its ability to provide knowledgeable care, using knowledge to bring a quality dimension to a period of a patient or client's life that would be unlikely to be achieved by a lay person. Caring is not the prerogative of nurses, there are many people who may provide care: 'it is the provision of professional, knowledgeable care that must identify the nursing profession' (Bishop, 2001). Nursing care may be very specific, such as is performed by specialist nurses, e.g. a dialysis nurse or an intravenous therapy nurse. However, much of general nursing practice is very diffuse, and identification of single interventions and judgement of their effectiveness is sometimes impossible with existing measuring

Table 3.1 *Influencing events for nursing 1966–2000*

Year	Event	Category
1966	Salmon Report	Management
1972	Briggs Report	Education
	Nursing Process	Practice
1977	Extended role of the nurse	Practice
1983	Creation of the UKCC	Education
1983	Griffiths Report	Management
1986	NVQ	Education
1988	Clinical Grading	Management
1990	Project 2000	Education
1991	Internal Market	Management
1991	Nursing Development Units	Research
1992	Multidisciplinary Audit	Practice
1992	Scope of Professional Practice	Education
1992–1995	Integration into Higher Education	Education
1995	Clinical Guidelines	Practice
1999	Nursing Strategy	Practice and Education
1999	Peach Commission (UKCC, 1999)	Education
2000	New pay structure due	Management

NVQ, National Vocational Qualification.
UKCC, United Kingdom Central Council for Nursing, Midwifery and Health Visiting.

instruments. There are so many other variables which cannot be controlled, such as the overall environment, other staff, family and so on. There is a view, which I share, that 'nursing must now face the reality that past professional strategies have denied it the power base in clinical practice it now requires to promote leaders who will remain in nursing practice and to have its voice heard in the clinical decision making process' (Kyzer, 1992). A career structure, which supports and maximizes the potential of nurses in clinical practice is now becoming a reality. The *Agenda for Change* (Department of Health (DoH) 2004, Royal College of Nursing (RCN), 2005) provides nurses within the NHS with details of how terms and conditions of service are determined, the relation between grades and pay bands and how career progression may be supported (see also Chapter 9 Useful addresses, page 121).

Never have nurses had more scope, such a breadth of areas in which to work, nor as much possibility for support. In 1992, the UKCC published *The Scope of Professional Practice* with the aim of providing the nursing and midwifery professions with the means to develop responsive and flexible health care services. *The Scope of Professional Practice* established the principle of extended roles for nurses and has facilitated the potential for nurses to determine aspects of their own role development. The undertaking of new roles and crossing traditional barriers requires nurses to demonstrate their competence and accountability. These important initiatives have shaped the current strategic Nursing and Midwifery Council (NMC) developments we have today, e.g. in relation to advanced nursing practice (see also Chapter 2).

Other forces driving forward changes have been policy driven, such as the reduction in junior doctors' hours (NHS Management Executive, 1991) and the imperative to have a primary-care-led NHS (NHS and Community Care Act 1990), which have had a significant impact on community-based staff (Jenkins-Clarke *et al.*, 1997). While in the view of Luker (1992) no-one was too sure what a 'primary-care led NHS' meant (a view more recently echoed by Ross (2000), who recognized that this presented opportunities for community nurses to consider new ways of working). Add to this rapidly changing NHS scenario the fact that the 'user' of the NHS has been very much at the focus, this often led to the development of nursing roles which had previously not been considered, where medical interventions were not needed but professional care was.

This does not mean that nursing has arrived in an ideal professional environment – the challenges are still there! However, the culture of change need not be seen as threatening, rather it provides a unique opportunity to embrace new ideas and create what Scott (2001) calls a 'let's have a go' mentality: in her view key to success in change is excellence in leadership at both clinical and managerial levels. One of the world's richest men, Bill Gates, said in a television interview that good leadership is about inspiring passion in colleagues. To have a passion for nursing is to embrace the challenges that accompany any demanding career and develop strategies to support the best of nursing care. Changing health needs and patterns of care offer unique opportunities, opportunities for the nurse–patient relationship to become stronger and less fragmented, for the nurse to offer care which is sensitive to the cultural needs of the patients, to really make care 'user centred'. Opportunities abound within the newly developing frameworks of care for health promotion and health education to come to the fore – an undervalued aspect of nursing which perhaps only health visitors have really taken forward to date.

Much of the success of any individual will depend on the vision and support of good management and careful career planning. What is so good now is that the combined efforts of members of various bodies, such as the nursing officers in the DoH, RCN, Unison and others have roles based in clinical practice as part of career advancement in nursing alongside education and management roles. These developments grew from the White Paper *The New NHS – modern and dependable* (DoH, 1997) and a second report, perhaps most useful for nursing, *Making a Difference* (DoH, 1999). Both make it clear how the government of the day was committed to extending developments in the roles of nurses. *Making a Difference* is an important platform to help the nursing professions to pursue a radical and progressive agenda (Moores, 1999). This is all set in the context of clinical governance (see below), and highlights the importance of research and development. The impact of clinical governance on nurses and the responsibilities attached to this are discussed below.

The creation of nurse consultant posts has brought further recognition of nursing expertise and attached higher salaries to these posts. Although some media reports have mocked this innovation, seeing it as a drop in the ocean, I share the view that we can only achieve the recognition, empowerment and concomitant funding for nursing care if we have advanced leading practitioners highlighting our work. These posts, if properly supported and filled by professional experts, will be the forerunners of the qualified nurses of the future, and we would all do well to watch their progress carefully. The key roles of modern matrons are designed to have a major impact on hospital cleanliness and reduction of the number of hospital-acquired infections.

Crossing professional boundaries and nurse-led services

There has been a move to develop nurse-led services, partly driven by the nursing profession and partly by a supportive DoH which is anxious to configure services to meet as many needs of the consumers as possible with a limited workforce. This is in part due to the reduction in junior doctors' hours (NHS Management Executive, 1991; Calman, 1993) and in part due to a need to move from the existing models of care, which have been traditionally medically focused, and provide a more patient-centred model of care, which is responsive to the specific needs of patients and clients. There are many nursing practices today which are either well established or are, with the new current ethos of collaborative partnerships, breaking across old barriers. A few examples which come to mind are: establishment of nurse-led clinics, collaboration of nurses with the police in the development of nurse-led assessment services at arrests, out-reach services for the socially excluded, NHS Direct (the nurse-led health helpline), and nurse-led walk-in centres.

These developments owe much to the work of Pearson and colleagues (1995) and later to the Sainsbury Family Trust funding of four nursing developments units (NDUs) based on the philosophy of Pearson and like-minded colleagues. Nursing development units are based on the concept of patient empowerment, clinical excellence, innovation and nurse leadership. Key features of an NDU funded by the DoH are shown in Box 3.1. The subsequent DoH-funded evaluation study is extremely useful reading for the student as there are many pertinent references to major policy initiatives that have impacted on the nursing profession over the past 10 years, not least *The Patient's Charter* (DoH, 1991), which was the precursor of the strong user focus currently being promoted.

Box 3.1 Nursing development unit

- Staff commitment to the NDU philosophy
- Clinical development: striving for excellence
- Evaluation of care
- Clinical nurse leadership: management support

The background to the NDU programme is well described by Vaughan (1998) and in the 'Master Class' by Redfern and Murrells (1998). The accompanying review by Bond (1998) highlighting the difficulties of research and audit is well worth the student's attention. It affords a unique opportunity to read open critique and response to peer review – the true test of a professional approach. The NDU initiative has had a major impact on nursing services, and has been adapted by many NHS trusts. At last, here was formal recognition of specific nursing expertise. Yes, nurses could and would break out of traditional moulds of task-oriented care and provide nursing which was open to change, centred on user perspectives, and based on willingness to work in a culture of inquiry. Such units are still running in many areas and they were certainly the forerunner of the numerous current diverse nursing initiatives. The recognition, stimulated by the NDU initiative, had a positive knock-on effect for clinical practice and a platform has developed which has established collaboration between higher education and clinical areas. In an important paper Read (1999) draws attention to the importance of proper management planning and support which is needed to underpin the provision of nurse-led services. Read has a record of research in this field and had developed the strong impression that nurse-led services often fail to reach their full potential, at least in part because of inadequate management. As the profession becomes more dynamic, and more complex, it is paramount that each individual nurse understands his or her own accountability and legal responsibilities (Glover, 1999).

Future developments

So how will health care look from a nursing perspective in the future? While a crystal ball would be handy, it is not needed to recognize that the focus, which is now on primary care, where previously it has been on hospital care, makes for many changes. Nurses working with general practitioners, currently the largest single group of nurses, are taking over many of the tasks previously carried out by doctors. This is not only in health promotion and triage, but also in running clinics, making referrals and prescribing. In the drive for seamless services hospitals are becoming less central and more specialist services have developed, such as rheumatology clinics, pain clinics and well people walk-in centres, many of which are nurse led. Although it cannot ever be economically viable to have centres of excellence in highly technical medicine with costly equipment in every locality, service beds for minor and general surgery will be available in smaller hospitals, many of them privately run. The 'integration' of the private sector with the NHS through the latter purchasing beds and services is a key development.

A great challenge for the immediate future is the increase in the older population, an increase that is unlikely to change as life expectancy becomes longer with healthier living and access to good health care. As families become less and less stable the effects on lone elders need to be carefully considered in health planning for the future. This is but one of the many challenges for the future, a future which will be determined by genetic engineering, advances in every area of technology, an increasing population overall, and, as far as one is able to judge without the crystal ball, depleted natural resources. The challenges presented by this or any similar scenario can only be won by working collaboratively – not only across health disciplines, but also with the general public, the users. The future of nursing lies in balancing expert knowledge with care, which is sensitive to the needs of the consumer.

The joys of achieving this balance, in terms of job satisfaction, the ability to provide and deliver the quality care which students are taught to give, will be more than repaid in terms of retention of staff, therapeutically enhanced patients and clients, and successful partnerships within the health care team. Historically, nursing has never appeared to be better placed to take forward a new professional status that will empower its practitioners to provide the care they are well equipped to give, to take their rightful place in society, at the bedside and at the policy table. This will not be achieved by innovation alone, however well publicized. This will only be achieved, in the long-term, by nursing continuing to show its reflective and dynamic abilities, and by sound research underpinning its practice.

Summary

A brief history is provided on the development of nurse-led services, and some examples have been given. While the difficulties in the creation of nurse-led services, which are not properly supported managerially, have been highlighted, the benefits in terms of improved patient/client care and staff satisfaction from successful implementation of new nursing roles have been stressed.

RESEARCH AND DEVELOPMENT IN NURSING

The importance of research and development in the NHS presents a major challenge to nurses. Why? Because without evidence, scientifically derived, to support nursing practice and to underpin standards, there are no criteria for care provision,

and no substantive arguments for qualified staff. In a medically dominated arena nursing research is at odds with the medical model and often penalized accordingly in terms of recognition and funding. This section highlights the progress to date and identifies the issues of particular importance to nursing practice. This is discussed in the context of clinical governance and clinical effectiveness. Issues specifically identified include utilization of research findings, understanding research, working for a research degree, and the usefulness or otherwise in professional terms, of achieving this. References are provided for further reading.

- What makes a good nurse?
- What is effective nursing?

A policy versus practice dilemma: Have you ever visited a relative or friend in a hospital and, as you arrive at the entrance to the ward thought 'This seems a good place' or 'Heavens, I wouldn't like to be a patient here!'? Most people of whom I ask this question know exactly what I mean. We are talking about a therapeutic environment. A good nurse contributes to that environment, as well as effectively carrying out his or her work. A poor nurse may still efficiently do their work but their effectiveness is less, or maybe even detrimental. Pearson (1998) stated that effectiveness can be achieved in the absence of excellence. Our challenge is to marry effectiveness and excellence. There is a plethora of initiatives to enhance nursing care and service delivery, with a particular focus on evidence-based practice. It is the view of Maggs (1997) and one which needs some exploration, that nursing staff are being asked to measure outcomes of care rather than to record the process of care, i.e. the quality of nursing and health care delivery. Donabedian (2003) stressed the equal importance of process with outcome. Much of nursing is process rather than an easily defined intervention so to disregard models of research, which ignore, because of the difficulty in measurement, the philosophical basis of nursing, is to disregard the activities of the largest health care workforce.

Student nurses are not expected to rush off and 'do research', but developing a questioning approach to practice, based on applying evidence, and watching and finding out what is going on is the beginning of developing research mindedness.

The major difference between research and a questioning approach is that research must always be disciplined and attempt to control everything that affects what is being studied. Reflective practice is a feature of the learning process and personal and professional development. It refers to the opportunity for nurses to reflect, and perhaps react, and learn from experiences. It is a feature of courses for nurses at all levels and encourages inquiry concerning practice, research application and analysis of nursing developments. This may lead to some modification of the nurse's original approach or a more advanced approach next time.

Evidence-based practice

DiCenso *et al.* (1998) define evidence-based practice as follows:

> In practising evidence-based nursing, a nurse has to decide whether the evidence is relevant for the particular patient. The incorporation of clinical expertise should be balanced with the risks and benefits of alternative treatment for each patient and should take into account the patient's unique clinical circumstances.

Deighan and Boyd (1996) offer the definition of a clinical learning strategy, and provide a substantial background to the development of evidence-based health care in this country, highlighting the strengths, and weaknesses of this approach to care provision. In a publication aimed at nurses, midwives and health visitors, the NHS Executive highlighted some of the benefits of clinically effective care such as improved consistency of care, shorter waiting lists and increased value for money (NHS Executive, 1998). Opponents of the evidence-based practice movement are concerned that it offers a 'cook book' approach to care with potential for rigidity. Whichever stance is taken in the debate, most agree that evidence-based care has a role to play in reducing variation. The issue of how you, the practitioner, are supposed to access all the available evidence for every patient or client is a vital one which deserves far more attention than is currently the case.

What is central to the nursing research agenda is the generation of a body of knowledge, which can underpin excellence in care, no small challenge given the limitations of available instruments! All registered nurses have the responsibility to apply up-to-date knowledge to practice.

Bridging the theory–practice gap

As a practice discipline, nursing shares with the other practice disciplines, such as medicine and social work, the difficulty that so much of its fundamental knowledge base originates from other disciplines, e.g. biology, chemistry, psychology. The 'gold standard' method of collecting research data has been considered by the scientific community generally to be the randomized controlled trial. This method employs a reductionist approach where the environment and all related variables are controlled. Clearly this cannot always be applied to nursing interventions. Nursing relies on patient experiences, personal and cultural contexts and relationships between patients and those who care for them (Maggs, 1997). Carr-Hill (1997) lists criteria that should apply to all research in terms of data quality, theoretical adequacy and policy relevance, and suggests that the dichotomy between quantitative and qualitative data is overplayed. However, research into social processes raises a number of dilemmas, one of which is the problem of subjectivity and its resulting bias (Mulhall *et al.*, 1999). Nursing research does much to promote understanding and clarity of practice-based issues and to generate evidence for nurses to use, share, and explain and promote appropriate standards of care.

It is beyond the remit of this chapter to take you through the fundamentals of nursing research, however, some texts are recommended for reading at the end of the chapter. What I have hoped to do is to raise an awareness of the issues that surround nursing research and to offer pointers for further study, if you wish. All nurses, however, should be research aware, as a matter of professional accountability, and to assist in this useful addresses are listed at the end of Chapter 9.

National Institute for Clinical Excellence

Establishing what constitutes 'best practice' is something of a political minefield, for what is deemed best from one perspective, or discipline, may not find agreement with another! When resources are limited, cost also plays a major part in any equation when defining best practice. Do you fund rare and highly costly treatments for a few, at the expense of treating a bigger population for a greater number of minor illnesses? Attention is being paid by the media to what is termed the 'postcode lottery' of health care. This is due to some health authorities funding more expensive treatments than others. The National Institute for Clinical Excellence (NICE) evolved in an attempt to neutralize some of these contentions and in response to the challenges presented to the health care professions, not least those establishing best practice and putting clinical governance into operation. However, as Freshwater (1999) points out, while a variety of available evidence is to be appraised, the scope of NICE is heavily weighted towards medical interventions, pharmaceutical practice, diagnostic techniques and procedures. It is thus of particular importance that nursing includes itself in the work of NICE, so that the profession is a player in the drive towards clinical governance (see Chapter 9 Useful addresses, page 121). Only nurses who have the education and confidence to cut through the jargon of health care research, to understand the key role that they play in health care provision, and be unafraid, open-minded and questioning in their approach to research can achieve this. Hence it is the responsibility of the registered nurse to understand research findings and to question practice.

SUPPORT FOR CLINICAL EXCELLENCE

In this section, the drive for a quality NHS, which meets users' needs, and supports staff in achieving this, is discussed. The role of clinical supervision, which will encourage the accountable individual nurse to develop his or her potential, and which will encourage the sharing of skills, successes and difficulties, is explained and its relevance to clinical governance demonstrated.

Quality and standard setting

The drive for a quality framework in the NHS was underpinned by Maxwell (1984) who was a major proponent in the UK of the work of Donabedian. However, whereas Donabedian focused equally on process, implementation and outcome, Maxwell and other proponents of 'quality' could be accused of forgetting the importance of process and of concentrating on outcome measures. For over 10 years 'outcomes' in terms of waiting lists, and any other indices which could be counted, have formed the basis of audit and quality. Maxwell described how the key elements which determined the quality of health care were relevance, accessibility, effectiveness, acceptability, efficacy and equity (cited in Marinker, 1994). These six elements were adapted for clinical audit, and although none of the health professions have a shared definition of audit (Kogan and Redfern, 1995) it is broadly interpreted as the measurement of professional activity which may be measured against predefined standards.

The former community health councils have now been replaced: consumers of health care services have their views represented at the local level and this relates to the NHS trusts.

Clinical supervision

The nursing professions have the responsibility of self-regulation; nurses who do not uphold the standards laid down can be removed from the NMC professional register. Clinical supervision, properly implemented, offers that opportunity to practitioners to develop their practice. It is about empowerment rather than control, though the term 'supervision' is off-putting to some, with connotations of management looking over your shoulder! This is NOT what clinical supervision is about. Clinical supervision had been practised in some pockets of enlightened nursing (mainly in mental health) but was first formally introduced to the nursing professions in the early 1990s. There are many definitions of clinical supervision including the following devised at a workshop on clinical supervision:

> Clinical supervision is a designated interaction between two or more practitioners, within a safe/supportive environment, which enables a continuum of reflective, critical analysis of care to ensure quality patient services.
>
> (Bishop, 1998a)

The components of clinical supervision are described in full elsewhere (Butterworth, 1996; Bishop 1998b; Fowler 2003). Clinical supervision is close in concept to mentorship and preceptorship, with the key difference being that the supervisor may not necessarily be senior but a peer or equal. Clinical supervision pulls together most of the concepts which have been discussed in this chapter so far. It embraces reflective practice, research and evidence-based practice, critical thinking, and is about life-long learning. It is about setting personal and shared standards in care giving and takes you, the practitioner into the centre of focus during that activity. You matter. So what are the goals of clinical supervision? Platt-Koch (1986) describes them as the expansion of the practitioner's knowledge base, assisting in the development of self-autonomy and professional accountability. The ultimate aim, of course, is to promote excellence in practice from supported and happy staff.

The perceived benefits of clinical supervision are well described by Kohner (1994) who studied five DoH-funded NDUs that had implemented clinical supervision. The benefits included enhanced patient care, professional growth with self-assurance and confidence, broadened thinking and improved relationships between all health care professionals.

The concept of 'clinical supervision' is not yesterday's notion – it is embedded in *Making a Difference* (DoH, 1999) and is pivotal to nurses making a real contribution in clinical governance. For this reason management must be committed to its success at every level. Clinical supervision is not a cheap option: it requires, time, budget, manpower and training. Supervisors must be trained, and in the view of some senior nurses who have implemented clinical supervision, supervisees should be trained as well. Certainly induction courses are needed, and the ethos of valuing staff promoted. Shared skills and a culture of caring critique will take nursing into this new millennium with unshakeable confidence and an ability to play its full part in the health care agenda.

Clinical governance

The concept of clinical governance was introduced *The New NHS* (DoH, 1997), and in the subsequent White Paper *A First Class Service – quality in the new NHS* (DoH, 1998). It is described as a framework through which NHS organizations are accountable for continuously improving the quality of their services and for safeguarding high standards of care by creating an environment in which excellence in clinical care will flourish. There are many nurses who are proponents of clinical governance, as it is seen to offer a unique opportunity for researchers and practitioners to work together – particularly at the point of care delivery – to maximize health care improvements (Boden and Kelly, 1999). It is the aim of clinical governance to draw together all these excellent mechanisms already in existence to support quality care from accountable staff. A professorial colleague of mine is tremendously enthusiastic and refers to clinical governance as 'the glue, which holds the best together, and provides the necessary transparency to see where improvements need to be made'. Scott (2001) describes clinical governance as a concept which is process driven not function-oriented, which puts the processes of care and the patient experiences at the heart of the new culture. Certainly it is clear that the development of clinical governance offers clinical nurses the opportunity to influence the clinical agenda within a trust, equals within a multi-disciplinary forum, which has not existed to date. Clinical governance, properly carried out, will put the power of the NHS back into clinical activity, rather than in the creation of layers of management and bureaucracy. Figure 3.1, taken from Scott (2001) expresses succinctly the key components of the clinical governance model.

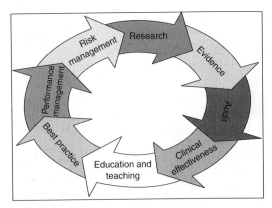

Figure 3.1 *The core elements of clinical governance create the basis for good care pathways (redrawn by permission of the publisher from Scott I (2001) Clinical governance. In: Bishop V, Scott I (eds) Challenges in Clinical Practice. Basingstoke, Palgrave Macmillan)*

Commission for Health Improvement

The Commission for Health Improvement (CHI) was established by the government to improve the quality of patient care in the NHS across England and Wales. The Commission has the brief to assure, monitor and improve the quality of patient care through clinical governance reviews. The CHI visits every NHS trust every four years. Its findings are based on evidence from the work of the trusts and how National Service Frameworks and NICE guidelines are being met at the local level.

Summary

Mechanisms to support the provision of quality care in the NHS are discussed in the context of nursing: quality frameworks, audit, clinical supervision and peer review, and clinical governance. Clinical governance aims to underpin the existing frameworks, and is seen to offer nursing an opportunity to demonstrate more openly its major contribution to health care services.

CONCLUDING THOUGHTS: NURSING FOR THE FUTURE

In drawing together all the issues raised in this chapter you will need to consider how best to offer individualized patient care within a hierarchy of care needs; look into the future and consider what shape nursing may need to take to meet the needs of society as a whole and nurses as a group. Questions of professionalism, elitism and pragmatism should run around your mind – it would be so interesting to know your thoughts at the beginning of your career.

Nursing in the UK has the wind of change behind it. Consider, in the light of the recent history, what permutations are likely for skill mix in an economy that is struggling to support an increasingly elderly population, and straining to keep up with the explosions in technology. Will we develop into an all-graduate profession in England as the other UK countries have done? What will identify the 'expert' nurse, and how best may the profession be represented at the policy table? Perhaps the leading question should be 'How can the NHS provide individualized patient care which is user centred, meets the demands of a knowledgeable and litigious society, in an economy which indicates little sign of expansion?' These are the real challenges to health care professionals.

Perhaps the contribution of nurses, who are the largest group of professional staff in the NHS, will be understood as the configuration of service change in response to users and career demands. Training and education programmes for student nurses are already involving patients and families; patients from ethnic minorities are rightly influencing our services to their communities; socially excluded individuals are at last beginning to be heard. This has a little to do with politics, and a great deal to do with the confidence with which our nursing profession is embracing such diverse agendas. The government has committed itself in *Making a Difference* (DoH, 1999), the national strategy for nursing in England, and has placed research highly in that portfolio. Whatever the national priorities are, it must be a priority of the profession to care for itself, to support each other and to share our undoubted expertise. If we support each other and base our knowledge on sound education and research we can meet any challenge.

REFERENCES

Bishop V (1998a) Clinical supervision, what is it? In: Bishop V (ed.), *Clinical Supervision in Practice: some questions, answers and guidelines.* Basingstoke: Macmillan.

Bishop V (1998b) What is going on? Results of a questionnaire. In: Bishop V (ed.), *Clinical Supervision in Practice: some questions, answers and guidelines.* Basingstoke: Macmillan.

Bishop V (2001) Professional development and clinical practice. In: Bishop V, Scott I (eds), *Challenges in Clinical Practice: professional developments in nursing.* Basingstoke: Palgrave, p. 78.

Boden L, Kelly D (1999) Clinical governance: the route to (modern, dependable) nursing research? *Nursing Times Research* 4, 177–88.

Bond S (1998) Masterclass. Review. *Nursing Times Research* 3, 289–90.

Briggs A (1972) Committee on Nursing. Cmnd. 5115. London: HMSO.

Butterworth T (1996) Primary attempts at research-based evaluation of clinical supervision. *Nursing Times Research* **1**, 96–101.

Calman K (chair) (1993) *Hospital Doctors: training for the future*. Report of the Working Group on specialist medical training. London: DoH.

Carr-Hill R (1997) Choosing between qualitative and quantitative approaches. *Nursing Times Research* **2**, 185–6.

Department of Health (1991) *The Patient's Charter*. London: HMSO.

Department of Health (1997) *The New NHS – modern, dependable*. London: The Stationery Office.

Department of Health (1998) *A First Class Service – quality in the new NHS*. London: DoH.

Department of Health (1999) *Making a Difference. Strengthening the nursing, midwifery and health visiting contribution to health and health care*. London: DoH.

Department of Health (2004) *Agenda for Change: what will it mean to you? A guide for staff*. London: DoH.

Deighan M, Boyd K (1996) Defining evidence-based health care: A health care learning strategy? *Nursing Times Research* **1**, 332–9.

DiCenso A, Callum N, Ciliska D (1998) Implementing evidence-based nursing: some misconceptions. *Evidence Based Nursing* **1**, 38–40.

Donabedian A (2003) *An introduction to quality assurance in health care*. Oxford: Oxford University Press.

Faugier J, Butterworth T (1994) Clinical supervision. A position paper. Manchester: Manchester University.

Fowler J (2003) Supporting practitioners in giving high quality care. In: Hinchliff S, Norman SE, Schober JE (eds), *Nursing Practice and Health Care*, 4th edn. London: Arnold.

Freshwater D (1999) Conference report: Taking responsibility for making a difference. *Nursing Times Research* **4**, 395.

Glover D (1999) Accountability. *Nursing Times Monograph*. London: Emap Publications.

Griffiths (1988) *Community care: agenda for action*. London: HMSO.

Jenkins-Clarke S, Carr-Hill R, Dixon P *et al.* (1997) *Skill Mix in Primary Care. A study of the interface between the general practitioner and the primary health care team*. York: York University.

Kogan M, Redfern S (1995) *Making Use of Clinical Audit: a guide to practice in the health professions*. Buckingham: Open University Press.

Kohner N (1994) *Clinical Supervision in Practice*. London: King's Fund.

Kyzer D (1992) Nursing policy; the supply and demand for nurses. In: Robinson J, Gray A, Elkan R (eds), *Policy Issues in Nursing*. Milton Keynes: Open University Press.

Luker (1992) *Health visiting: towards community health nursing*. Oxford: Blackwell.

Maggs C (1997) Research and the nursing agenda. Confronting what we believe nursing to be. *Nursing Times Research* **2**, 321–2.

Marinker M (1994) *Controversies in Health Care Policies. Challenges to practice*. London: BMJ Publications.

Maxwell RJ (1984) Quality assessment in health. *BMJ* **288**, 1706–8.

Moores Y (1999) Making a Difference – the foundation for a future ripe with opportunity. *Nursing Times Research*, **4**.

Mulhall A, LeMay A, Alexander C (1999) Bridging the research – practice gap: A reflective account of research work. *Nursing Times Research* **4**, 119–30.

NHS and Community Care Act 1990. London: The Stationery Office.

NHS Executive (1998) *Achieving Effective Practice. A clinical effectiveness and research information pack for nurses, midwives and health visitors*. Leeds: NHS Executive.

NHS Management Executive (1991) *Junior Doctors: The new deal*. London: NHSME.

Pearson A (1995) A history of nursing development units In: Salvage J, Wright S (eds), *Nursing Development Units; A force for change*. Harrow: Scutari Press.

Pearson A (1998) Excellence in care: Future dimensions for effective nursing. *Nursing Times Research* **3**, 25–7.

Platt-Koch LM (1986) Clinical supervision for psychiatric nurses. *Journal of Psychological Nursing* **16**, 982–6.

Read S (1999) Nurse-led care: The importance of management support. *Nursing Times Research* **4**, 408–21.

Redfern S, Murrells T (1998) Masterclass. Research, audit and networking activity in nursing developments units. *Nursing Times Research* **3**, 275–88.

Ross F (2000) Commentary. The challenges ahead for public-health nursing. *Nursing Times Research* **3**, 193.

Royal College of Nursing (2005) *Agenda for Change. A guide to the new pay and conditions in the NHS*. London: RCN.

Salmon (1966) *Report of the Committee on Senior Nursing staff structure*. London: HMSO.

Scott I (2001) Clinical governance. In: Bishop V, Scott I (eds) *Challenges in Clinical Practice*. Basingstoke: Palgrave.

United Kingdom Central Council (1992) *The Scope of Professional Practice*. London: UKCC.

United Kingdom Central Council (1998) Paper to inform developments of the specialist practice framework, the assessment of competence. London: UKCC.

United Kingdom Central Council (1999) *Fitness for Practice*. The UKCC Commission for Nursing & Midwifery Education. (Chairman Sir Leonard Peach) London: UKCC.

Vaughan B (1998) The story of NDUs – How the nursing, midwifery and health visiting development unit programme began. Masterclass. *Nursing Times Research* **3**, 272–4.

FURTHER READING

Baly MA (1995) *Nursing and social change*, 3rd edn. London: Routledge.

Rolf G, Freshwater D, Jasper M (2001) *Critical Reflection for Nurses and Health Care Professionals: a user's guide.* Basingstoke: Palgrave.

Bishop V (ed.) *Clinical Supervision in Practice. Some questions, answers and guidelines.* Basingstoke: Macmillan/ NTresearch.

Johns C, Freshwater D (1998) *Transforming Nursing through Reflective Practice.* Oxford: Blackwells.

Atkinson T, Claxton G (2000) *The Intuitive Practitioner.* Buckinghamshire: Open University Press.

Bishop V, Scott I (eds) *Challenges in Clinical Practice.* Basingstoke: Palgrave.

4

Perspectives on Adult Nursing

Penny Harrison

INTRODUCTION

The aim of this chapter is to discuss the role of the 'adult nurse' within health care and their contribution to the health of adult patients. Links with health studies and the other three branches of nursing and the range of placements where students of adult nursing may gain experience will be explored. Some key nursing activities that may be experienced by an adult patient will also be discussed.

To take a closer look at adult nursing it is necessary to review some key concepts that assist in defining health care and nursing. Henderson (1966) (cited in Aggleton and Chalmers, 2000) stated that all individuals have social, spiritual, biological and physical needs as human beings, and these needs are shared by all people. Henderson also stated that nursing is about assisting an individual, sick or well, in the performance of activities that contribute to health, recovery from illness or peaceful death. These activities are performed in such a way as to maximize the individual's potential or actual level of independence.

Fatchett in 1998 stated that a new agenda is now making its presence felt in nursing, and in the UK this is linked to the modernization of the National Health Service (NHS). These are challenging nursing to change its traditional perspectives and move to a professional model of organization, which includes:

- patients as active participants in their care
- the nurse as health educator
- care is patient-focused, not task-focused
- appreciation of patients' holistic needs
- co-operation and collaboration with other health care services.

Adult nurses form the largest group within professional nursing as a whole, therefore these changes are likely to be far-reaching for all nurses caring for adult patients across a variety of settings including primary care, acute care and social care.

ADULT NURSING

As stated in the introduction, nursing may be defined as the diagnosis and treatment of human responses to actual or potential health problems (*Medical, Nursing and Allied Health Dictionary*, 2002). The nurse uses four key points of reference in the definition or underpinning framework of nursing care. These are the phenomena of nursing itself, theories to observe for nursing interventions, planning nursing actions, delivering and evaluating the care relative to those activities.

Nursing adult patients requires study of a wide range of subjects related to health and health care as well as developing practical nursing skills. Theory is usually learnt in the classroom, but is related to practical nursing and then applied to real patients in the clinical placement settings. Naidoo and Wills (2001) have suggested that these subjects are collectively known as health studies (summarized in Box 4.1).

Although these subjects relate to all types of nursing, adult nursing has its own unique aspects of care. Alexander *et al.* (2000) see adult nursing as assisting individuals to maintain good health, to recover from episodes of illness, to cope with aspects of chronic health or disability and to have a dignified end to life. Adulthood is usually taken to start at mental and physical maturity. This can mean that boundaries between nursing adolescents

Box 4.1 Subjects in health studies

- Anatomy and physiology
- Epidemiology
- Psychology
- Sociology
- Cultural studies
- Social and health policy
- Management studies
- Health economics
- Ethics
- Legal aspects of care
- Health promotion

Source: Naidoo and Wills (2001)

Reflective activity

Look at the subjects listed in Box 4.1. Do you know what they all mean? Reflect on why they might contribute to the study of health care.

and adults can be blurred. In clinical practice, nursing adults is usually taken to mean caring for individuals who are aged 18 years and over. Thus an adult nurse will receive education and training in skills that will equip them to nurse adult individuals in a variety of practice settings such as the individual's home, community settings, day-care centres, clinics, health centres, a general practice or hospital or specialist facilities, for example hospices.

Adult nursing offers a wide and varied choice of career opportunities in the settings mentioned above, within or outside of the NHS, as well as a range of work within these settings. Adult nurses may be involved directly or indirectly in four key areas of work (Box 4.2).

Box 4.2 Adult nursing: key areas

- Clinical practice
- Education
- Research
- Management

Reflective activity

Reflect on your work in a previous health care setting or currently with your clinically based mentor. What aspects of the care that you have delivered to your group of patients reflected one or more of the key areas of nursing identified in Box 4.2?

The adult nurse's scope of practice is wide-ranging, and this is one of the strengths of adult nursing. No two days are ever the same. No two patients have exactly the same needs. Each day brings chances to learn new skills, practise existing skills and gain a wealth of knowledge, professional and interpersonal qualities. The adult nursing student develops many skills including problem-solving, using evidence and research findings to enhance patient care as well as reflective skills to review the progress made. There are many opportunities to develop practice in a huge variety of areas and specialties. These may be focused in wards, clinics or community settings.

Some adult nurses choose to become teachers of nursing. This may be within a formal setting such as a university or may be based within the practice area itself focusing on a range of staff from nursing auxiliaries, to qualified practitioners or students of nursing. Some adult nurses have a role within formal research programmes or trials. Other nurses may be using research skills in other roles, for example, the ward-based nurse may also be using research or evidence about practice within their day to day work. Experienced nurses may also be managers of staff or teams. For some this may be as a ward sister or nurse manager. Adult nurses have many transferable skills that lend themselves to a variety of managerial roles within nursing as well as more widely within the NHS. Dowding and Barr (2002) suggest that qualified adult nurses use a range of management skills within their daily working lives to organize their work and those of the team within which they are based to assess, plan, deliver and evaluate the care for the patients within their charge.

Recently, there has been a range of developments within nursing. Although these may also apply to educational setting and 50 per cent within clinical practice areas. During training, the student is assessed through their assignments, case studies and exams. In clinical practice, the student is assessed by their mentor with a practice book being completed to demonstrate competency.

Within clinical practice a formally nominated **mentor** supports the adult nursing student. A mentor is an experienced nurse who acts as a role model, guide and facilitator of learning for the student for the duration of their placement. The mentor would have undertaken formal training, usually with teaching in clinical-practice-based skills and would be familiarized with the programme that is delivered by the local school of nursing. Some mentors have taken formal teaching courses to develop their skills in relation to teaching students within clinical practice.

Placements

Placements vary in length of time, but since the publication of the United Kingdom Central Council's (UKCC) *Fitness for Practice* in 1999 the emphasis has been on longer rather than shorter placements, frequently of up to eight or 12 weeks' duration. This is to allow the students to settle within the area, develop their confidence and gain the best learning opportunities from the area. Mentors spend a minimum of 40 per cent of their time with students. In many clinical placement areas this figure may be higher. In other areas, in the absence of the nominated **lead** mentor, another qualified nurse or **associate** mentor supports the student. This individual will continue the work and learning opportunities planned by the student and lead mentor.

The benefits of working with mentors for the duration of the placement are continuity and consistency of the learning opportunities afforded within the placement. The benefit of working with an associate mentor for parts of the clinical placement allocation may include variety in learning opportunities, as well as exposure to another qualified nurse. In some instances the associate mentor may be a relatively newly qualified nurse, though not usually within the first six months of initially qualifying. The benefits of having an associate mentor who has qualified recently will be that the experience of being an adult nursing student has not been forgotten.

Thus there may be common experiences and empathy to be shared between the student and associate mentor, and sharing of the learning which may be two-way between the student and their associate mentor. This is also true of the relationship between the student and their lead mentor. Whereas the lead mentor will have experience, possibly from a variety of clinical settings over some years, the student will bring a questioning approach to the clinical environment or sometimes new ideas or research findings that can be shared. Confident mentors will harness the shared skills and experiences of the adult nursing student plus their own skills to develop competent practice in the student as well as having the benefit of updating and maintaining their own personal and professional development.

Placement settings are varied and encompass a wide range of areas. Nurses who are responsible for developing nurse education within practice may also use a rotation between related areas. Examples of some placement settings are given below in Box 4.4.

Box 4.4 Examples of placement setting

A **Within primary care**
- General practitioner surgeries
- Health care centres
- District nursing
- Walk-in health centres
- Minor injuries units
- Specialist disabled or rehabilitation units
- Community hospitals
- Nursing homes

B **Within an acute hospital**
- Accident and emergency departments
- Assessment wards
- Medical wards
- Surgical wards
- Rehabilitation wards
- Specialist medical wards, e.g. neurological medical ward
- Specialist surgical wards, e.g. ear, nose and throat surgical ward

- Out-patient clinics
- Specialist areas, e.g. burns/stroke units
- Operating theatres and recovery rooms
- Critical care areas, e.g. intensive care/coronary care/high dependency units

C Within other areas
- Hospices
- Private hospitals
- Specialist services, e.g. alcohol rehabilitation programmes
- Undertakers
- NHS Direct

Gaining the best from placements

The new placement can seem a daunting experience. The student may well have experience of a range of shifts, perhaps from a health care setting or work experience from another environment or profession. Adult nursing students of nursing can expect to work a variety of shifts/shift patterns. These may include day as well as night shifts, working at weekends and holiday periods. The variety of shifts is immense so a summary is included here (Box 4.5).

Box 4.5 Examples of shift times

8-Hour shifts
- Morning/early shift – 07:00 to 15:00 hours
- Afternoon/late shift – 14:00 to 22:00 hours
- Night shifts – 21:00 to 08:00 hours

12-Hour shifts
- Day shift – 07:15 to 19:45 hours
- Night shift – 19:15 to 07:45 hours

Shift for work with a specialist nurse
Usually eight hours anytime between 07:30 to 19:00 hours

The student can expect to be shown around and orientated to the placement area at commencement of the experience. This is likely to include layout and location of emergency equipment such as the resuscitation trolley, fire exits, etc. During

the first week of the placement the student usually has the opportunity of an informal interview with their mentor. This is to outline the learning opportunities available and set goals and action plans to achieve the objectives. This may also be an opportunity for the mentor to plan rotation between the different areas related to the placement setting. This will be to ensure the student sees the patient group that they will meet throughout all the areas available. An example of this is given below in Box 4.6. Many placement areas have a nurse responsible for organizing the student nurses' placements, both in terms of shifts to be completed, nomination/allocation of mentors and rotation programmes. An information book may also supplement this. Often this is sent to students prior to their arrival within the area. The benefit of this is to allow students to have information about their forthcoming clinical placement area prior to arrival.

Box 4.6 Example of a rotation programme for an adult surgical ward

- Pre-assessment clinic
- Admission to surgical ward
- Following patient through from ward to operating theatre/recovery
- Working with specialist nurses during patient's recovery, e.g. nutrition nurse specialist
- Discharge planning
- Out-patients

Reflective activity

Think about the area in which you are gaining clinical experience at the moment.

What areas link or relate to the group of patients that you are caring for? List the related areas. Ask your mentor to arrange for you to visit or work with the linked areas.

dependence, the term *essential* has been used to emphasize the importance of these aspects of care. This is set out in the document *Essence of Care* (DoH, 2001). This is due to their relationship of essential aspects of care on long term health and recovery from episodes of ill health. These essential aspects of care are just as important as some of the more technical aspects of nursing care such as the recording of the patient's vital signs such as blood pressure, pulse, temperature. Binnie and Titchen (1999) suggest that such essential aspects of care are 'practical' nursing skills and should not be given lightly to untrained or junior staff. This is because they form part of the unusually privileged access to patients and remain central to nursing's function.

CONCLUSION

Fatchett (1998) stated that nurses have developed a range of new skills that will assist them to work within the modernized environment that forms the NHS today. Research/evidence-based care, quality, auditing, standard setting and benchmarking skills, health promotion/education plus care protocols and multi-professional/collaborative working practices are all features of modern nursing. For adult nursing this is likely to be particularly challenging. Adult nurses already work in busy, pressurized environments. Walsh (2000) suggests that there is now a shift away from the scientific and technological paradigm as the sole option for the caring professions, and that the cost of caring is more valuable to patients than the cost of giving this care to the nurse. Thus if adult nursing is to meet the challenges it will require combining the best of traditional nursing skills as well as the continuing development of newer styled skills.

GLOSSARY

In the context of this chapter the meanings of the following words are described:

Anatomy and physiology	Study of the structure (anatomy) and the function (physiology) of the body
Best practice/evidence-based practice	Nursing practice based on evidence to support the nursing care/interventions. Research may be used as evidence to show that a particular aspect of care is effective for the adult patient
Biology	Study of living organisms and their products
Clinical mentor	Named qualified nurse whose role is to facilitate learning and who assesses the student in the clinical practice setting
Clinical placement	Area where a student nurse works with their clinical mentor to learn the art and science of nursing
Clinical skills	Skills used in practice, e.g. giving an injection or dressing a wound
Cognitive skills	Developing skills of reasoning, critical thinking
Diagnosis	Identification of a disease or evaluation of signs and symptoms
Dietician	Qualified health care practitioner providing assistance with the management of nutrition and food
Disease	Specific disease or disorder characterized by a set of recognizable signs and symptoms
Epidemiology	Study of disease/disease events in populations
Ethics	Study of moral values or principles
Handover	Transfer of information from one group of nurses to another
Health care	Provision of services by health care professionals/practitioners to prevent, maintain or manage a state of health
Health promotion	Health education programmes/information designed to improve, maintain or safeguard health for individuals or the community
Motor skills	Physical skills
Multi-professional team	Team of qualified health care practitioners and support staff working together to deliver patient care
Nursing	Nurse assisting in the care and treatment of activities of living and/or human responses to actual or potential health problems

Nursing interventions	Acts or actions by nurses to implement plans of care for patients
Occupational therapist	Qualified health care practitioner who helps patients to develop skills to cope with physical, social or emotional deficits
Pharmacist	Qualified health care practitioner who assists with the formulation, dispensing and advice regarding drugs or medication to the multi-professional health care team, patient or their carer
Physiotherapist	Qualified health care practitioner concerned with the physical examination, testing and treatment of physical impairments through a range of techniques including exercise
Psychology	Study of behaviour and the mind
Reflective practice	Thoughtful review of one's actions
Social worker	Qualified health care practitioner who deals with social, emotional and environmental problems that may impact on a patient's health
Sociology	Study of people and societies
Symptoms	Indication of a disease or disorder

REFERENCES

Aggleton P, Chalmers H (2000) *Nursing Models and Nursing Practice*, 2nd edn. Hampshire: Palgrave.

Alexander M, Fawcett J, Runciman P (2000) (eds) *Nursing Practice. Hospital and home: the adult*, 2nd edn. Edinburgh: Churchill Livingstone.

Baillie L (2001) (ed) *Developing Practical Nursing Skills*. London: Arnold.

Binnie A, Titchen A (1999) *Freedom to Practice: the development of patient-centred nursing*. Oxford: Butterworth Heinemann

Department of Health (1999) *Making a Difference. Strengthening the nursing, midwifery and health visiting contribution to health and health care.*London: DoH.

Department of Health (2000) *The NHS Plan*. London: The Stationery Office.

Department of Health (2001) *Essence of Care – benchmarking and audit tool kit for essential aspects of care.* London: The Stationary Office.

Dowding L, Barr J (2002) *Managing in Healthcare: a guide for nurses.* Harlow: Prentice Hall.

Ellis R, Betts M (2002) *The nurse as a communicator.* In: Kenworthy N, Snowley G, Gilling C (eds) *Common Foundation Studies in Nursing*, 3rd edn. Edinburgh: Churchill Livingstone.

Fatchett A (1998) *Nursing in the New NHS: modern, dependable?* London: Bailliere Tindall.

Henderson V (2000) In: Aggleton P, Chalmers H (2000) *Nursing Models and Nursing Practice*, 2nd edn. Hampshire: Palgrave.

Medical, Nursing and Allied Health Dictionary, 6th edn. St. Louis: Mosby, 2002.

Naidoo J, Wills J (2001) (eds) *Health Studies: an introduction.* Hampshire: Palgrave.

Nursing and Midwifery Council (2000) *Guidelines on Administration of Medicines.* London: NMC.

Nursing and Midwifery Council (2004a) *Standards of Proficiency for Pre-registration Nursing Education.* London: NMC.

Nursing and Midwifery Council (2004b) *The NMC Code of Professional Conduct: standards for conduct, performance and ethics.* London: NMC.

United Kingdom Central Council (1999) *Fitness for Practice.* London: UKCC.

Walsh M (1998) *Models and Critical Pathways in Clinical Nursing: conceptual frameworks for care planning.* London: Bailliere Tindall.

Walsh M (2000) *Nursing Frontiers: accountability and the boundaries of care.* Oxford: Butterworth-Heinemann.

Watson N, Wilkinson C (2001) *Nursing in Primary Care.* Basingstoke: Palgrave.

ANNOTATED FURTHER READING

Aggleton P, Chalmers H (2000) *Nursing Models and Nursing Practice*, 2nd edn. Hampshire, Palgrave. An effective text that reviews the various models of nursing used within a variety of practice settings.

Alexander M, Fawcett J, Runciman P (2000) (eds) *Nursing Practice. Hospital and home: the adult*, 2nd edn. Edinburgh: Churchill Livingstone. A comprehensive text that reviews the principles and practices of adult nursing. Relevant to nursing students and for the newly qualified practitioner. Highly recommended.

Cormack D (2000) (ed) *The Research Process in Nursing*, 4th edn. Oxford: Blackwell Scientific. An effective text introducing nursing students to the research process.

Dimond B (2005) *Legal Aspects of Nursing*, 4th edn. London: Prentice Hall. A thorough review of legal aspects of nursing and implications for clinical practice.

Dougherty L, Lister S (2004) (eds) *The Royal Marsden Manual for Clinical Nursing Procedures*, 6th edn.

Oxford: Blackwell Scientific. A procedure manual including care plans for many aspects of nursing care and interventions. Highly recommended.

Dowding L, Barr J (2002) *Managing in Healthcare: a guide for nurses.* Harlow: Prentice Hall. Principles of the management of nursing care are reviewed within this text.

Hinchliff S, Norman S, Schober J (2003) (eds) *Nursing Practice and Healthcare.* 4th edn. London: Arnold. A comprehensive text reviewing principles of nursing practice.

Maslin-Prothero S (1997) (eds) *Study Skills for Nurses.* London: Bailliere Tindall. A text that assists students to develop study skills for both pre-registration nursing courses and for post-registration studies.

Medical, Nursing and Allied Health Dictionary, 6th edn. St. Louis: Mosby, 2002. Many dictionaries are available. This one is comprehensive.

Naidoo J, Wills J (2001) (eds) *Health Studies: an introduction.* Hampshire: Palgrave. Principles of health promotion explored within this text.

Seeley R, Stephens T, Tate P (2003) *Anatomy and Physiology.* 6th edn. Boston, McGraw Hill. A comprehensive anatomy and physiology text that is specifically designed for nursing. Appropriate for both pre-registration and post-registration students.

Smeltzer S, Bare B (2000) *Brunner and Suddarth's Textbook of Medical-Surgical Nursing,* 9th edn. Philadelphia: Lippincott. A comprehensive text that reviews the principles and practices of adult nursing. Relevant to nursing students and for the newly qualified practitioner.

Trounce J (2004) *Pharmacology for Nurses,* 17th edn. Edinburgh: Churchill Livingstone. A comprehensive text that reviews the principles of pharmacology for nursing. Relevant to nursing students and for the newly qualified practitioner. Highly recommended.

Walsh M (1997) (ed.) *Watson's Clinical Nursing and Related Sciences,* 5th edn. London: Bailliere Tindall. A comprehensive text that reviews the principles and practices of adult nursing. Relevant to nursing students and for the newly qualified practitioner. Highly recommended.

Watson N, Wilkinson C (2001) *Nursing in Primary Care.* Basingstoke, Palgrave. A text that reviews the principles and practices of nursing adults within primary care settings. Relevant to nursing students and for the newly qualified practitioner.

USEFUL WEBSITES

Nursing and Midwifery Council. www.nmc-uk.org
Department of Health. www.open.gov.uk/doh/dhhome.htm
Royal College of Nursing. www.rcn.org.uk
National Institute for Clinical Excellence. www.nice.org.uk

JOURNALS RECOMMENDED FURTHER READING

British Journal of Community Nursing
This journal focuses on nursing within primary care and the interface between acute care, primary care and social care.

British Journal of Nursing
A peer-reviewed journal with a range of articles relevant to adult nursing within a range of clinical settings. This journal is particularly effective at presenting nursing research in an understandable and accessible format.

Nursing Standard
This is published by the Royal College of Nursing. A range of news, views and peer-reviewed articles of interest to adult nurses. Widely available in many high street outlets.

Nursing Times
Britain's most widely read journal that consists of about one-third news articles, one-third clinical articles, with a large recruitment/job advert section. Again, widely available throughout the UK.

Professional Nurse
A professional and readable journal that focuses on developing nursing care and clinical practice, which reflects evidence-based care, quality initiatives and the modernization agenda.

Nursing Times and *Professional Nurse* are now one journal.

917 755 5976

917 011 5976 5976

917 755 755

917

5

Perspectives on Children's Nursing

Kevin Power

INTRODUCTION

The aim of this chapter is to provide an insight into children's nursing. The key ideas and philosophies underpinning children's nursing will be explored to aid understanding of the world of children's nursing. Aspects of the course content and clinical experiences will be discussed to provide guidance on how to get the most out of a course. The principal sections of this chapter are:

- Historical insights into children's nursing
- Child health policy affecting children's nursing
- An outline of children's nursing
- Why sick children need children's nurses
- Making the most of the Common Foundation Programme
- Starting in practice
- How to get the most out of a placement
- Essential skills in children's nursing
- Sources of knowledge and information

Children's nursing is a popular choice of study and many courses are oversubscribed. At the interview, course applicants are usually expected to show some insight into children's nursing. It can be very difficult, if not impossible, to gain experience in children's nursing prior to commencing a pre-registration nursing course. There are relatively few opportunities to become employed as a health care assistant (HCA) and many hospitals apply age restrictions on anyone wishing to undertake work experience from school on a children's ward. Thus, many students embarking on the child branch of a nursing course may have little idea of what children's nursing is like or what it involves.

This chapter therefore aims to help develop that insight which will help enhance any application to a children's nursing course. It is also aimed at introducing those who may already have secured a place on a course to some of the main issues that will impact on their practice.

It is important to recognize that children are different from adults and have different care needs. As we shall see later in this chapter children experience different illnesses and respond to some illnesses differently than adults. For example a simple cold in an adult could be a serious respiratory infection for a young child. Therefore this chapter also provides an outline some of the different needs children have in health care and the skills the nurse requires to meet these needs.

HISTORICAL INSIGHTS INTO CHILDREN'S NURSING

Dr Charles West recognized that children needed specialist care when ill and in 1852 he founded the Great Ormond Street Hospital for Sick Children in London. He then established training programmes specifically to prepare nurses in the care of sick children (Miles, 1986). In 1919 the Nurses Registration Act established the requirement for nurses to be entered on a national register (Parker, 1996). A separate professional register was created for children's nurses, although according to Whiting (2002) this was to prevent children's nurses masquerading as general nurses rather than as a recognition that children need specially trained nurses to care for them.

In 1989 the first Diploma of Higher Education and BSc (Hons) courses in nursing began and those graduating from these courses were qualified in adult, mental health, learning disabilities or children's nursing. The courses consisted of an 18-month **common foundation programme** (CFP) and an 18-month **branch programme**, specializing in one of the four branches of nursing. Following a review of nursing education in 1999, the former United Kingdom Central Council for Nursing, Midwifery and Health Visiting (UKCC, now the Nursing and Midwifery Council (NMC) made recommendations (UKCC, 1999) that led to the current situation of a one year CFP and a two-year branch programme. The four branches of nursing remained the same as before.

Debates have taken place regarding the future of the separate branches of nursing (UKCC, 2001; Whiting, 2002) although no definite action has been taken as yet. Thus it can be seen that the children's nursing education has undergone, and is likely to continue to undergo, changes that reflect current thinking. Many of these changes are influenced by child health policies originating from central government.

CHILD HEALTH POLICY AFFECTING CHILDREN'S NURSING

The organization of children's health care is determined by policy set at government level and many reports and studies have influenced the policy changes. Laws such as the **Children Act 1989**, the **Human Rights Act 1998** and the **Protection of Children Act 1999** also influence children's nursing practice and education. It should also be noted that although the Children Act 1989 itself only directly relates to those children defined as 'in need', the principles within the Act are applied to the care of all children. One of these principles is that of Parental Responsibility. Only those with parental responsibility are able to give consent for a child to undergo examination or treatment. Policy and law does change over time and therefore it is important for children's nurses to be aware of these changes when they occur. An example of this is a change in the legal definition of when a father may have parental responsibility

for a child. The **Adoption and Children Act 2002** made an alteration to the original definition laid down in the Children Act 1989. From December 2003 fathers who were not married to the mother at the time of the birth may automatically have parental responsibility if they are named as the father on the birth certificate (Adoption and Children Act 2002 (Commencement No. 4) Order 2003 section 2.2 (a)).

Unfortunately, tragedies also inform policy such as that detailed in the **Victoria Climbié Inquiry** report (Laming, 2003). Additionally, the adoption of international conventions by the UK government, such as the **United Nations Convention on the Rights of the Child** (UN, 1989), also influence children's nursing. The most recent initiative determining child health services in the National Health Service (NHS) involved the **Children's Taskforce**, set up by the Department of Health (DoH), creating a national set of standards called the **Children's National Service Framework** (NSF) (Box 5.1). This framework sets new national standards across the NHS and social services for children.

Box 5.1 The Children's National Service Framework

The framework is an important way of responding to some of the key challenges facing children's health and social care services, for example:

- Responding to *Learning from Bristol: the report of the public inquiry into children's heart surgery at the Bristol Royal Infirmary 1985–1995*
- Mainstreaming the successes of programmes such as Quality Protects and Sure Start
- Most importantly, the Children's NSF will be about putting children and young people at the centre of their care, building services around their needs.

Source: DoH (2002a)

The first part of the NSF for children was published in 2003 by the DoH and this set out the standards for the provision of services for children in acute hospital settings. Three key standards are set out in the NSF:

- services should be centred around the needs of children
- care must be of high quality and based on good evidence
- the hospital environment should be safe and appropriate for children.

The third key challenge identified for the NSF, and the first standard in the NSF, points to one of the central themes in children's nursing: that of seeking out and taking seriously children's views regarding their care when planning care. This is also reflected in the Children Act 1989 and the UN Convention on the Rights of the Child 1989, and is embodied in the Human Rights Act 1998. A number of other themes or ideas underpin children's nursing practice and these will be considered in more detail further on in this chapter.

Summary

- Nurses Registration Act 1919 established a register for nurses with a separate register for children's nurses.
- Ongoing debates regarding the future of children's nursing as a separate branch.
- Children's views about their own care a key principle in children's nursing.
- NSF recognizes a need to design services specifically for children.

AN OUTLINE OF CHILDREN'S NURSING

If a survey of children's nurses were to ask 'What is a children's nurse?' there are likely to be many different answers. The reason is that children's nurses practise in a wide variety of areas and specialities (Box 5.2). Therefore it is difficult to pin down exactly what children's nursing is and what a children's nurse does, and a simple description of a children's nurse's work would not do the role justice. Clearly a children's nurse could not hope to practise effectively across all these specialities and in all areas of practice. This means

that children's nurses may focus on a particular area such as surgery and may then specialize into a particular type of surgery such as ear, nose and throat surgery. Others may work mainly with adolescents or work in the community caring for children with chronic or long-term illness at home or working in a children's hospice. What this does reveal is the potential for a children's nurse to develop a career in many different and varied areas of care.

Box 5.2 Examples of areas of practice and specialities in children's nursing

- Hospitals
- Medical wards
- Surgical wards
- Orthopaedics
- Ear, nose and throat
- Oncology (cancer wards)
- Out-patients clinics
- Accident and emergency
- Operating theatres
- Out-reach services, e.g. specialist respiratory nurses providing some care in the child's own home
- Neonatal units (for premature babies)
- Intensive care
- Community
- Child's own home
- Schools
- Special schools, i.e. schools for children with special mobility needs or a learning disability
- Young offenders institutions
- Health promotion such as advising parents and children on healthy diets or dental hygiene, or providing sexual health information for adolescents
- Mental health care such as helping young people deal with emotional problems or such serious issues as anorexia and bulimia

In addition to the many areas of practice that a children's nurse might work in, increasingly opportunities are becoming available to acquire a specialist practitioner qualification that is recognised by the NMC. Ultimately there is the potential for the children's nurse to become a consultant nurse. Alternatively there are opportunities to develop a career in leading nursing through management or becoming a researcher. Essentially registering as a children's nurse following three years of hard work need only be the first step in a wide and varied career in children's nursing.

Notwithstanding all the different areas of practice the majority of what is written about children's nursing suggests that there is an underlying philosophy or set of ideas about what children's nursing is. This philosophy is evident in a Royal College of Nursing (RCN) statement (RCN, 1992) about the principles underpinning all their policies regarding child health (Box 5.3).

Box 5.3 Principles underpinning children's nursing

- Recognize each child as a unique, developing individual whose interests are paramount
- Listen to children, attempt to understand their perspectives, opinions and feelings, and acknowledge their right to privacy
- Consider the physical, psychological, social, cultural and spiritual needs of children and their families
- Respect the right of children, according to their age and understanding, to appropriate information and informed participation in decisions about their care

Source: RCN (1992)

It can be seen that within the RCN philosophy statement, in common with the UN Convention on the Rights of the Child (UN, 1989) and the Children Act 1989, that the issue of children's rights is a significant feature of children's nursing practice. Within the UN Convention, three main rights underpin all the others and these must be taken into account in any decision relating to or affecting children.

1 All the rights in the Convention apply to all children equally whatever their race, sex, religion, language, disability, opinion or family background (Article 2)
2 When adults or organizations make decisions which affect children they must always think first about what would be best for the child (Article 3)
3 Children too have the right to say what they think about anything which affects them. What they say must be listened to carefully. When courts or other official bodies are making decisions which affect children they must listen to what the children want and feel (Article 12)

These three rights are also evident within the Children Act 1989 and firmly established within UK law through the Human Rights Act 1998. Thus it is clear that the principles of equality, best interests and the right to participate in decision-making are central to the care of children.

Another key value or principle underpinning children's nursing is that of **family-centred care**. Coleman (2002) suggests that family-centred care is an evolving concept that is influenced by changes in society and the health care system. There are several views in the literature about how to define family-centred care and this is evidence that it is an evolving concept. Nethercott (1993) argued that family-centred care has seven critical components. Although there are some drawbacks to viewing family-centred care using Nethercott's list (Smith et al., 2002) each of the seven components she outlined will be explored here as they do provide an easily digestible description of the main elements of family-centred care.

1 The family must be viewed in its social, cultural and religious context.

At times of stress, family members should not be required to conform to norms that are alien to them. This means that the care should be organized as far as possible to fit the 'normal' pattern of the family. There are limits to this of course. It would be impossible to arrange different mealtimes for each individual child in a hospital or organize community children's nurse visits purely to suit individual families.

2 The roles of individual family members must be evaluated to help meet their physical and emotional needs and to maximize their individual roles in providing care for their child.

about

child + family

It would be incorrect to assume that parents are always the main carers for a child. Grandparents or even older sisters or brothers may fill this role in some families. Therefore the nurse must ascertain the role fulfilled by each member of the family especially in relation to the care of an ill child.

3 Information should be explicit to enable participation in decision-making and the acquisition of knowledge pertaining to their child's illness.

This means that the nurse should be giving information to families and children in a manner that the lay person can understand. Much of the information used by professionals concerning a child's care is expressed in jargon or technical words that are not part of everyday language.

4 The prime caregiver should be involved in developing and evaluating care plans.

The prime caregiver for the child is the person who normally cares for the child at home. This means that the nurse becomes an advisor rather than the person who decides alone what care is given and when. The nurse must use his or her knowledge to guide and assist the family in making plans of care and should not merely dictate what they feel should be done.

5 The involvement of families in technical aspects of care should be in accordance with their own perceived ability and willingness to develop the necessary skills.

The nurse may be able to teach family members how to carry out technical aspects of the child's care. Care needs to be taken, however, to ensure that no pressure is put on the family to be involved in the care of a child if they do not wish to or feel they lack confidence. Sometimes it is just as important for the family to get a rest as it is for the child to be given care.

6 Usual childcare practices, unless detrimental to the child's well-being, should be continued in hospital.

There may be a number of ways of caring for children and professionals may prefer some of these as opposed to others. However, families have to make their own decisions about how to care for their children and some of these choices may not coincide with the view of professionals. For example, breast milk is generally recognized as best for infants but bottle-feeding may be the family's preferred option.

7 The impact of the sick child on the family should be evaluated and steps taken to ensure support continues as needed after discharge or in the event of death.

Research has shown (Callery, 1997) that having a sick child in hospital or at home can have significant social and financial impact on families. It is important that any problems in these areas are identified and alleviated as much as possible.

Reflective activity

Having read Nethercott's main or key components of family-centred care, make a list of the qualities or skills the children's nurse should exhibit to make family-centred care work.

Some of the skills and qualities you thought of may be listed in Table 5.1. Do not worry if you did not think of all of these. There will be, no doubt, some qualities that you have thought of that have not been included in the table.

These are some of the essential personal skills and qualities that a children's nurse should develop to deliver family-centred care. Having thought about what skills and qualities might be required by a children's nurse let us now consider some of the reasons why children should be cared for by children's nurses.

WHY SICK CHILDREN NEED CHILDREN'S NURSES

Child disease

Some people believe that children are essentially small adults and thus do not need nurses specifically educated to care for them. This is far from the truth, not only do children grow, their bodies are also developing. That is to say that the way their bodies work is different in many respects from an adult. This means that a child's physiology changes over time until eventually they have the same characteristics as adults. During this time many differences are apparent that the children's nurse needs to take account of. For example, children's total daily fluid requirements change with age and

Table 5.1 *Critical attributes of a nurse enabling family-centred care*

Qualities and skills	Reason for children's nurse having the quality or skill
Be an informed, flexible practitioner	Able to give clear and easily understood information to families
Evidence-based practice	Ensure that any advice or information given is up to date and the best available
Able to adapt to different care delivery	Able to adapt hospital routines to fit families' needs
Not see nursing as a source of power, but accept parents as partners in care	If families' needs are to be cared for they need to become equal partners in their child's care
Nurses should be advisors but should accept that advice may be ignored	Parents need to make their own decisions about what is best for their child. (There may be some exceptions to this where a child's health or life is threatened)
Nurses need to actively listen to families	Families can only become true partners in care if their views are listened to and taken seriously
Be able to manage without the security offered by routines and hierarchy	Set routines may be fine for the nurse but they do not fit with a family's usual patterns of care
Have mature and refined interpersonal skills and self-awareness	Nurses must be expert communicators and these are essential key skills in communication
Need to be skilled in asking the right questions, listening to answers, helping the family to understand	If the right questions are not asked how can the nurse know what the family's needs are and how best to cater for them?
Have knowledge of theories related to the family and of the processes, which influence family functioning	Essential for the understanding of different families and their different needs

weight and thus the nurse needs knowledge of these changes to ensure a child is receiving sufficient fluids for their needs. This is especially the case when children develop illnesses that cause fluid loss, such as diarrhoea and vomiting, which is relatively common in young children.

As a child grows, the amount of any particular drug that they may be prescribed needs to be altered in response to changes in the child's weight. Children's nurses must therefore be adept at calculating the appropriate dosage of any drug according to the child's weight. This will prevent over or under dosage both of which can be detrimental to the child's continued good health.

Children's diseases are different from adults: see Table 5.2 for a comparison of the commonest reasons why people ring NHS Direct for health advice for children and adults. In addition children respond differently to the same diseases that adults may also experience. For example, most fit adults cope relatively well with a respiratory tract infection, such as a cold. However a young child has much narrower air passages than an adult, and any infection that causes inflammation or swelling

Table 5.2 *Ten commonest symptoms on which advice was sought from NHS Direct in 1999[1] (National Statistics, 2000[2])*

Children	Adults
Fever	Abdominal pain
Rash	Headache
Vomiting	Fever
Diarrhoea	Chest pain
Cough	Back pain
Abdominal pain	Vomiting
Cold/influenza	Breathing difficulty
Headache	Diarrhoea
Head injury	Urinary symptoms
Ingestion (includes overdose and poisoning)	Dizziness

[1] Based on information collected monthly from 13 NHS Direct sites between April and September 1999.
[2] Source: Department of Health. Crown copyright material is reproduced with the permission of the Controller of HMSO and the Queen's Printer for Scotland.

in the child's air passages will cause a more significant degree of respiratory distress. This is because the child has less 'spare capacity' in the air passages to cope with the narrowing that occurs in response to the swelling. Thus an infection that may cause symptoms of a cold in an adult can lead to severe breathing problems in the young child. Indeed, the commonest reason for admission to hospital for children is respiratory problems (DoH, 2002b). Children's nurses thus need to be vigilant for signs of respiratory distress when caring for children with respiratory infections. Very young children are also unable to tell a nurse when they are having difficulty breathing, so being able to identify the outward signs of respiratory distress becomes a particular skill for the children's nurse.

Children are also still developing their ability to think, use language and understand the world around them. This is termed **cognitive development**, and this must be borne in mind when communicating with and caring for children. Taylor *et al.* (1999) have outlined some of the implications of cognitive development on the children's nurse:

- Under 2s can best be communicated with via their parents.
- Under 7s are less able to see the links between medical treatment and cure and may see unpleasant treatments as punishment for some misdeed.
- Under 7s find it difficult to have a concept of the internal workings of the body. They can only appreciate what they can see and experience.
- Over 12s can begin to imagine the implications of chronic illness and sinister implications of pain.

Always check a child's level of understanding before embarking on giving any information. Be aware of the implications of certain words before using them with children, e.g. 'cut', 'destroy', 'remove'. Children over 7 years may appreciate the use of analogies such as 'baddies' for germs and 'goodies' for body defences but children under 7 years may take these terms too literally so check their understanding first.

It is clear then that the needs of children change as they develop and the children's nurse needs to be aware of these changes and how to adjust care activities and communication strategies to suit. It also needs to be recognized that **adolescents** have particular needs as they emerge from childhood into adulthood. The children's nurse may need to assist the adolescent and their family to understand the changes that occur and the particular needs that become apparent during this period.

Summary

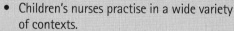

- Children's nurses practise in a wide variety of contexts.
- Children's rights are central to children's nursing.
- Three key rights for children are: equality of rights; best interests; listening to the child's views.
- Care for children should be centred on the family.
- Children are different from adults and have different health care needs due to their stage of development.
- Children respond differently to certain conditions/illnesses.
- Children understand the world in a different way than adults.
- Children's nurses must learn to communicate effectively with children from birth to adulthood.

Let us now consider how a student can make the most of the learning opportunities presented in the various parts of the pre-registration nursing courses.

MAKING THE MOST OF THE COMMON FOUNDATION PROGRAMME

The CFP aims to equip all students of nursing, regardless of which branch they intended to study, with the skills, knowledge and understanding that are common to all areas of nursing. This necessarily means that the content is generic in nature, that is to say applicable to all clients groups. For example, effective communication skills are central to nursing in all spheres and there are very many ideas and skills associated with communication that apply to the care of children as much as adults. Clearly there may be specific skills associated with caring for children as outlined previously. Similarly, essential nursing skills such as safe moving and handling of patients, first aid, assisting a person to bath and dress are required by all nurses. The principles underlying all these skills apply equally whether it is children or adults who are being cared for.

Social policy and sociological concepts or ideas are often incorporated into CFP learning and this can seem to have little to do with children's nursing. However as can be seen from the opening section of this chapter, government policies have a significant impact on the way children's services are delivered. Thus an understanding of where these policies come from and how they may be formulated is very important for a children's nurse. Indeed nurses need to demonstrate that they are fit for purpose (NMC, 2002). This means that nurses must be able to respond to the changing needs of the health services (NMC, 2002) and a knowledge of health and social policy is essential for this responsiveness.

It is not necessarily very easy when your motivation is towards children's nursing to appreciate perspectives on care from other disciplines. This is especially the case if you have no previous experience in children's nursing and are desperate to begin caring for children and their families. The CFP can seem to be a long wait for the first contact with your chosen area of nursing. However, the learning of caring skills and competencies is essential as a baseline for developing an understanding of children's nursing. Reflecting on the content and experiences of the CFP with other students and academic staff and thinking about how the knowledge and skills gained can be used in caring for children is an important aspect of a student's personal development within the course.

STARTING IN PRACTICE

It is a daunting prospect for most students to think of their first few days and weeks on a children's ward. How are you going to survive? One of the issues that students say they are worried about, for example, is being asked a question by a parent or child and answering the phone. In fact many students report that, after a period in practice placements, most of the questions that parents ask are fairly straightforward to answer and relate to the environment of the ward rather than technical questions regarding their child's care. It is helpful then to try to find out the answers to the questions that might be asked and thus be prepared beforehand.

> ### Reflective activity
>
> *Imagine that you are the parent of a 5-year-old child who has been admitted to hospital for the first time. Try to think of the questions you may have about the admission.*

You may have thought of issues such as the location of the toilets, where to get a cup of tea/something to eat, how to call for assistance, can you stay with the child, can I bath/shower my child, what are the rules about watching television. There may be a host of other practical questions that are probably very similar to the questions a student has when they first start on a hospital ward or a placement in the community. Thus if the answers to such questions are established in the first few days of placement parents' questions can be answered with more confidence.

However, there may be a myriad of other questions that children and families may ask, for example when their child can have a drink, go home, when may they re-start school. There is no shame for the student to admit he or she does not know the answer. It would be unreasonable to expect anyone new to an area to be able to answer all the questions a child and family may ask. The best response in these situations is to be honest and say 'I don't know, but I will find out for you [or get a more senior member of staff to help].' Even the most senior nurses may not be able to answer all the questions a family may have, therefore students should not feel that they must have the answers. In fact being asked a question that one does not know the answer to can prompt discovery of the answer and add this to one's own knowledge.

Community placements can also create feelings of anxiety for students. These feelings are often related to the unfamiliarity of the environment and being unsure what one is allowed to do and what not. This is particularly so when children are visited in their own homes. Students often report feeling inadequate or like a 'spare part' when accompanying **clinical mentors** in community settings. It is important to recognize that it is normal to feel somewhat out of place in what for the student is an unfamiliar environment. Observing the practitioner and noting the interactions between the child, family and practitioner is an important part of the learning process in community placements.

HOW TO GET THE MOST OUT OF A PLACEMENT

The primary responsibility of nursing staff is to care for the children and families. Therefore they do not necessarily always have time to think through what a student might need to learn or experience while in their area. This is especially the case since most areas will have students at differing stages of the course and even on different courses. This can make it difficult for clinical staff to be fully aware of each individual student's needs in terms of clinical learning. Thus the student who is well prepared, with an understanding of the learning outcomes specified for the placement, and able to inform their clinical mentor of what activities they wish to focus on to achieve these will be in a good position to negotiate meaningful clinical experiences. For example, if a learning outcome for a module specifies that the student should be able to assist in carrying out a nursing assessment, the student should mention to the clinical mentor that he or she wishes to observe an experienced nurse carrying out such an assessment. Then the clinical mentor can inform other staff that if they are admitting a child they should invite the student to observe. The student for their part can make it their business to know when a child is to be admitted and seek out the admitting nurse and request permission to observe. If there are particular **clinical nursing skills** that the student needs to practise then this is something to highlight with the clinical mentor.

Summary

- CFP aims to equip students with skills, knowledge and understanding of nursing common to all areas of care.
- Students should not be afraid to admit they do not know something.
- Practice placements provide opportunities for a great deal of learning.

- Students should take responsibility for their own learning.
- Ask lots of questions.
- Try not to accept what others say on trust, always ask for reasons why something is being said.
- Set personal objectives for learning in placements.
- Develop good relationships with the clinical mentor.

ESSENTIAL SKILLS IN CHILDREN'S NURSING

It would be impossible, in this text, to list all of the clinical nursing skills that should be learnt to be fit for practice as a staff nurse. The skills that should be learnt will range from day-to-day tasks such as making beds and administering medicines to the complex skills of teaching children and families how to continue care following discharge. Several texts are available outlining the range of clinical skills needed by children's nurses and guidelines on the delivery of those skills (Lawrence, 1998; Barber et al., 2000; Huband and Trigg, 2000). Most children's nursing areas/teams will also have nursing guidelines that outline a wide range of clinical skills and the standards expected in carrying these skills out. These nursing skills also need to be delivered to children of all ages and stages of development from infants to adolescents. This is because children of different ages and stages of development have particular needs in relation to various care activities. Taking a throat swab from an infant, for example, will involve techniques different from those required when doing the same with a toddler or an adolescent.

However, it needs to be acknowledged that it is not possible to learn every skill that a qualified nurse might need in the course of clinical practice. This is partly because there may not always be the opportunity to practise every skill during a pre-registration course. Learning new skills and refreshing existing skills continues after registration and throughout a professional nursing career. Nonetheless it is necessary to be able to demonstrate

competence in those nursing skills that enable the achievement of the competencies (NMC, 2002) for entry to the register of nurses. The NMC uses the term competence to describe 'the skills and ability to practise safely and effectively without the need for direct supervision' (NMC, 2002 p. 9). These competencies are designed to ensure the nurse can give and direct the safe and effective delivery of nursing care, including wider skills such as the ability to work effectively in a multidisciplinary team ensuring there is seamless delivery of care between the community and hospital teams. The children's nurse, working with adolescents who have chronic conditions or long-term care needs, will also require skills in facilitating a smooth transition for the adolescent from children's health care services to adult services at the appropriate time.

Contrary to appearances most children, both well and ill, are cared for in their own homes by the family, sometimes with the support of a children's nurse or other health professional specializing in the care of children. Generally speaking children are only admitted to hospital when they cannot be cared for at home. It is widely accepted in children's nursing that children are best cared for in the familiar environment of their own home. Therefore it is likely that there will be placements in the course with either some or all of the following:

- Health visitor
- School nurse
- Community children's nurse
- Children's outreach nurse
- Specialist health visitor

A significant range of skills need to be learned in the community. The nurse may be caring for a child in their own home and be more of an advisor and guide than a direct giver of care. Communication skills are particularly important to facilitate good quality care for the child. Being able to listen and take seriously the wishes of the family in relation to how the child is cared for is an important skill. If the child and family feel their views are taken into account it is more likely that they will respect the opinions of the nurse advising them. It follows then that learning to negotiate care effectively is an essential skill that can be observed in community placements.

In the community the family are likely to be giving the bulk of the care thus the opportunities for delivering direct 'hands-on' care may be limited. However where hands-on care is given by the nurse in the child's home particular consideration needs to be given to how any task might be completed. The environment may be less under the control of the nurse as he or she is a visitor in the home. Any supplies or equipment needed to provide care must be in the home already or taken in by the nurse. It is different from being in a hospital where if something is forgotten or not available on the ward it can be found from somewhere else. Thus there is a different emphasis on what is being learnt during community placements and this should be borne in mind when negotiating learning experiences with a clinical mentor in community placements.

Wherever the student is placed for learning experiences there are always likely to be challenging or difficult situations to deal with. It is important therefore to identify some of these and suggest ways in which they may be dealt with.

Emotionally challenging situations

Fortunately death is a rare occurrence in children's nursing except in intensive care areas, and even then it is not an everyday occurrence. Most children who are going to die do so in their own home. Even those who are cared for in a hospice tend to go home to be with their family in familiar surroundings prior to their death. It is important to realize that it is acceptable to get upset and to even shed a tear or two. The families will also realize that you are human and not an unemotional robot (White, 1995). There are times when a child will die unexpectedly and these are probably the most emotionally challenging times in a nursing career. It is important to recognize when the grief felt personally reduces the ability to effectively support the family. If this occurs it is best to let the clinical mentor or the senior nurse present know and withdraw from the situation. Qualified children's nurses are acutely aware that these are very difficult situations for students and will often spend as much time comforting students and helping them to come to terms with what has happened as they do with the family. Often the team will meet after the event and discuss feelings about what happened. It is important that students join in these discussions. It is essential that any feelings about the death of a child are shared and not bottled up inside as this will reduce the prospect of being able to deal with a similar situation in the future. In time it is possible to learn how to develop coping mechanisms that allow the nurse to effectively care for the family and at the same time show their own emotions without detriment to the ability to care.

Similar skills need to be developed with more common situations such as the child admitted in severe pain or who is critically ill. The essential difference in these situations is that often the nurse can do something to ease the child's pain or relieve the symptoms. Thus, while the child in pain is a distressing sight a great deal can be done to alleviate the pain. The critically ill child can be frightening to deal with at first but with experience the confidence in one's ability to care for the child grows and there can be a great feeling of satisfaction from providing care. The important fact to bear in mind is that the student is not alone and a qualified nurse should be on hand to assist. The student may feel they are not much help in these situations but it must be remembered that all qualified nurses were once in a similar situation, and with time and experience skills are developed that enable almost any situation to be effectively managed.

There are not just the emotional demands of children's nursing to consider but also the physical demands. Nursing is a physically demanding job as much of the day is spent on one's feet and it is possible to walk several miles in the course of a shift. This is especially the case in areas where children need to be escorted to other departments within a hospital. There are also the shift patterns to consider particularly if the student is not used to shift work. It can be demanding completing a late shift, going home and not being able to get to sleep because one is still 'buzzing' with the activity of a busy shift and then having to get up for an early shift the next day. As a result of this it is important to keep physically fit and look after oneself especially in the early days of the course. This is particularly important in view of the fact that the student is likely to be exposed to a great variety of infectious children, especially in the winter months.

Summary

- A vast range of skills need to be developed as a nurse ranging from the seemingly mundane bed-making to the highly complex teaching children new skills to enable then to care for themselves.
- Skills acquisition continues after qualification.
- The NMC set specific competences to be achieved prior to registration (see Appendix 1).
- Different skills may be learnt in hospital and community placements.
- Learning to cope with emotionally difficult situations is an essential skill for children's nurses.
- It is important to maintain personal fitness to be able to deal with the physical and emotional demands of the job.

SOURCES OF KNOWLEDGE AND INFORMATION

Throughout the course and indeed during the rest of a career as a nurse there is a need to ensure the most up-to-date information is used to gain or develop knowledge. **Journals** are usually the best source of the latest information because they are published on a regular basis. A number of journals that carry information, articles and research relating to children's nursing are available in or through most nursing libraries. Some of these will be specialist children's nursing journals, whereas others will be general nursing journals that have articles on or research reports relating to children's nursing and health care.

Specialist children's nursing journals

Journal of Child Health Care
This is the journal of the Association of British Paediatric Nurses and is published four times a year.

It has peer-reviewed articles written in a style and level similar to that required for academic essays.

Journal of Neonatal Nursing

This is published every two months, and it is a specialist journal for neonatal nursing publishing research articles. It provides information relevant to placements in neonatal areas.

Professional Care of Mother and Child

Largely a midwifery journal but it has a good number of peer-reviewed articles of interest to children's nurses.

Paediatric Nursing

This is a Royal College of Nursing journal, published monthly. It has news items and peer-reviewed articles on policy and practice. There is also a useful reference list of recent research and some critical reviews of recent research reports.

Archives of Diseases in Childhood

This is a medical journal with many articles relating to care and treatment of childhood illnesses. Many research articles relate to recent medical advances. It is not an easy read for the beginner. A fetal and neonatal edition is also published.

General nursing journals

British Journal of Nursing

This is a general nursing journal with regular children's nursing supplements. It frequently has articles relating to professional issues such as the law and professional conduct, and many peer-reviewed articles.

British Journal of Community Nursing

District nursing and health visiting are the main focus of this journal but regular articles on children's issues do appear.

Community Practitioner

This is the journal of the Community Practitioners and Health Visitors Association. Similar to the above.

Journal of Clinical Nursing

A general nursing journal focusing on research into clinical care. Regular children's nursing focused reports are included. It has mostly-peer reviewed articles.

Nursing Standard

General weekly journal published by the Royal College of Nursing. It has lots of news concerning nurses, some clinical articles and a few peer-reviewed articles.

Nursing Times

This is also a general weekly journal with lots of news concerning nurses. Similar to above.

Journal of Advanced Nursing

This journal is published fortnightly. It has peer-reviewed research reports, some of which are related to children's nursing. It also carries useful literature review articles. Not easy reading for the beginner.

Although the journals listed above are likely to contain a good deal of the information and knowledge needed throughout the course there are many other useful journals that should not be ignored. It is essential that children's nursing students recognize that even those journals that do not have a specific focus on children's health care are a useful resource.

CONCLUSION

It is important to remember throughout the course and on qualifying that it is not possible to be an expert nurse after three years on the course. The pre-registration nursing courses are designed to enable a qualified nurse to:

- assess a child's needs
- plan care based on those needs
- give or direct the giving of that care
- evaluate the effectiveness of that care and take appropriate action.

The course should provide a broad base for any nursing career and thus a great deal has to be learnt in the first few years of practice on qualification. The message then is clear. Be realistic regarding what can be achieved as part of the course. It is not necessary to learn everything and no-one should expect a newly qualified nurse to know everything. It is sufficient to be able to practise safely as part of a whole team in providing good quality care to children and their family in a variety of settings. Use every available opportunity to learn and get the most out of each placement.

Not all placements will be completely enjoyable experiences and students cannot like or be liked by everyone. Try to use the less than excellent experiences as a learning experience to identify what could have been done to improve the situation.

The most important aspect of children's nursing is to enjoy the learning and the children. It will be hard work at times but ultimately worthwhile. The rewards of helping children return home on the road to recovery outweigh the hard work and unsocial hours. There is also the prospect of a long and fruitful career with many opportunities to develop in clinical practice, education, research or management that make the hard work worthwhile.

GLOSSARY

In the context of this chapter the meanings of the following words are described:

Clinical mentor	A named qualified nurse whose role is to facilitate learning and assess the student in the practice setting.
Clinical skills	Skills used in the practice of nursing, for example giving an injection or dressing a wound.
Cognitive development	Development of the ability to think, reason and understand the world.
Evidence-based practice	Nursing practice based on evidence to support that practice. Research may be used as evidence to show that a particular nursing care is effective for a child. Child and/or family preferences may also be used to show that a particular nursing intervention should be used.
General nursing journal	Journal that carries articles relating to all areas of nursing including children's nursing.
NHS Direct	A 24-hour nurse advice and health information service for the public, providing confidential information on: what to do if you or your family are feeling ill; particular health conditions; local health care services, such as doctors, dentists or late-night-opening pharmacies, self help and support organizations (NHS Direct, 2003).
Orthopaedics	Literally means 'straight child'. This term refers to surgery to either

	correct some deformity of the bones or treatment for a break or fracture which may or may not involve surgery.
Peer-reviewed articles	Articles that have been read and checked for accuracy and relevance by an 'expert' in the field. Thus the conclusions drawn in such articles are likely to be better informed and more reliable than mere opinion.
Quality Protect	Three-year programme launched in 1998 by the UK government that set quality targets for the provision of children's services by local authorities.
Sure Start	Government initiative involving agencies at local and national level working together in new ways to improve services for young children under 4 years of age from disadvantaged areas and their families.

REFERENCES

Adoption and Children Act (2002) (Commencement No. 4) Order 2003. London: The Stationery Office.

Barber J, Campbell A, Morgan L (eds) (2000) *Clinical Care Manual for Children's Nursing*. Quay: Dinton.

Callery P (1997) Paying to participate: financial, social and personal costs to parents of involvement in their children's care in hospital. *Journal of Advanced Nursing* 25:746–52.

Coleman V (2002) The evolving concept of family centred care. In: Smith L, Coleman V, Bradshaw M (eds) *Family-Centred Care. Concept, Theory and Practice*. Houndmills: Palgrave.

Department of Health (2002a) www.doh.gov.uk/nsf/children.htm (accessed 21 March 2002).

Department of Heath (2002b) www.doh.gov.uk/HPSSS/TBL_B12.HTM (accessed 10 May 2002).

Department of Health (2003) *Getting the right start: National Service Framework for Children. Standard for Hospital Services*. London: The Stationary Office.

Huband S, Trigg E (2000) *Practices in Children's Nursing: guidelines for hospital and community*. Edinburgh: Churchill Livingstone.

Lawrence C (1998) Essential skills for paediatric nurses. *Paediatric Nursing* 10:6–8.

Laming L (2003) *The Victoria Climbié Inquiry*. London. The Stationery Office.

Miles I (1986) The emergence of sick children's nursing. *Nurse Education Today* 6:82–7.

National Statistics (2000) *Social Trends 30*. London: The Stationery Office.

Nethercott S (1993) A concept for all the family. Family-centred care: a concept analysis. *Professional Nurse* 8:794–7.

NHS Direct (2003) Welcome to NHS Direct Online. www.nhsdirect.nhs.uk/index.asp (accessed 22 December 2003)

Nursing and Midwifery Council (2002) *Requirements for Pre-registration Nursing Programmes*. London: NMC.

Parker E (1996) Development of paediatric nursing. In: McQuaid L, Huband S, Parker E (eds) *Children's Nursing*. Edinburgh: Churchill Livingstone.

Royal College of Nursing (1992) *Paediatric Nursing. A Philosophy of Care. Issues in Nursing and Health*. London: RCN.

Smith L, Coleman V, Bradshaw M (2002) Family-centred care: a practice continuum. In Smith L, Coleman V, Bradshaw M. (eds) *Family-Centred Care. Concept, theory and practice*. Houndmills: Palgrave.

Taylor J, Muller D, Wattley L, Harris P (1999) *Nursing children: psychology, research and practice*, 3rd edn. Cheltenham: Stanley Thornes.

The Adoption and Children Act 2002. London: The Stationery Office.

The Children Act 1989. London: HMSO.

The Human Rights Act 1998. London: The Stationery Office.

The Protection of Children Act 1999. London: The Stationery Office.

United Kingdom Central Council (1999) *Fitness for Practice*. London: UKCC.

United Kingdom Central Council (2001) *Fitness for Practice and Purpose: The Report of the UKCC's Post-Commission Development Group*. London: UKCC.

United Nations (1989) Convention on the Rights of the Child. New York: UN.

White C (1995) Life crises for children and their families. In: Carter B, Dearmun A (eds) *Child Health Care Nursing: concepts, theory and practice*. Oxford: Blackwell Science.

Whiting M (2002) Children's nursing education: towards consensus. *Paediatric Nursing* 14: 26–9.

ANNOTATED FURTHER READING

Carter B, Dearmun A (eds) (1995) *Child Health Care Nursing: concepts, theory and practice*. Oxford: Blackwell Science. This British book examines in some detail the key concepts that underpin nursing practice using examples from practice. There are some sections examining specific disease processes but the main focus is on the principles of care that can be transferred into almost any nursing situation.

Heath S (1998) *Perioperative Care of the Child*. Salisbury, Mark Allen. A relatively small and easily digestible book specifically focusing on the care of children and families before and after surgery.

Huband S, Trigg E (2000) *Practices in Children's Nursing: guidelines for hospital and community*. Edinburgh: Churchill Livingstone. A comprehensive guide to clinical skills in children's nursing. This very useful British text also includes rationale and literature sources to support the guidelines. Offers insights into community as well as hospital clinical skills. Useful introductory chapter on key concepts in children's nursing.

Moules T, Ramsey J (1998) *The Textbook of Children's Nursing*. Cheltenham: Stanley Thornes. A British children's nursing book that provides a comprehensive guide to practice.

Smith L, Coleman V, Bradshaw M (2002) (eds) *Family-Centred Care. Concept, theory and practice*. Houndmills: Palgrave. A useful text that explores in detail one of the key underpinning principles in children's nursing. There are a number of case scenarios and case studies to help the reader understand the issues that are being discussed.

Taylor J, Muller D, Wattley L, Harris P (1999) *Nursing Children: psychology, research and practice*, 3rd edn. London: Chapman and Hall. This is a useful text considering in some detail the psychological and emotional development and care of children. Some very useful critiques of current theories of child development that provide helpful material for assignments are included.

Hockenberry M, Wilson D, Winkelstein M, Kline N (eds) *Wong's Nursing Care of Infants & Children*, 7th edn. St Louis: Mosby. This comprehensive American text is now in its seventh edition. A highly respected book that covers virtually all one might wish to know about children's nursing. There are two drawbacks to note regarding this book. First, it is American and a number of things about American nursing practice differ from British nursing and these need to be borne in mind. Allied to this is that the language, drugs, equipment and clinical measurements used in the books do differ in some cases from Britain. The second drawback is the relatively high cost of the book.

As with all books that one is considering purchasing rather than borrowing from a library it is best to borrow first. If you feel comfortable with the way the text is laid out, the level of sophistication of the language and the scope of information offered then buy it. However it is worth remembering that books can go out of date because they are not able to update as rapidly as a journal that is published on a regular basis.

USEFUL WEBSITES

Association of British Paediatric Nurses. www.abpn.org.uk/ – contains useful information plus references for articles from back issues of the *Journal of Child Health*. There is also a link to the electronic version of the journal.

Action for Sick Children. www.actionforsickchildren.org/ – action for Sick Children is the UK's leading children's health care charity, specially formed to ensure that sick children always receive the highest standard of care possible.

www.internurse.com/ – this is an extensive internet resource for nursing with links to many articles references and scholarly papers plus news on the current debates in nursing.

http://nmap.ac.uk/ – this internet resource for nursing provides searching facilities for finding a wide range of information on all nursing topics.

www.jiscmail.ac.uk – this internet discussion group can offer stimulating debate on current issues in children's nursing and a resource for information. Two forums are particularly worth joining: Paediatric Nursing Forum and Child Health.

Royal College of Nursing. www.rcn.org.uk/index.php – the RCN website provides access to a wide range of information, resources and the students discussion forums. There is also a range of paediatric nursing forums at the RCN although membership of the RCN is required to access these.

USEFUL ADDRESSES

Action for Sick Children
C/O National Children Bureau
8 Wakley Street
London EC1V 7QE
Tel: 020 7843 6444

Association of British Paediatric Nurses
Norman Long Membership Secretary
c/o School of Nursing and Midwifery
De Montfort University
266 London Road
Leicester LE2 1RQ

Royal College of Nursing
RCN Headquarters
20 Cavendish Square
London W1M 0AB
Tel: 020 7409 3333
Fax: 020 7647 3425

RCN Welsh Board
Ty Maeth King George V Drive East
Cardiff CF14 4XZ
Tel: 029 2075 1373
Fax: 029 2068 0726
E-mail: welsh.board@rcn.org.uk

RCN Northern Ireland Board
17 Windsor Avenue
Belfast BT9 6EE
Tel: 02890 668236
Fax: 02890 382188
E-mail: ni.board@rcn.org.uk

NHS Careers
www.nhscareers.nhs.uk/index.html
Tel: 0845 60 60 655

6

Perspectives on Mental Health Nursing

Ben Thomas and Robert Tunmore

INTRODUCTION

The purpose of this chapter is to introduce students to contemporary mental health nursing as a career option. The incidence of mental illness will be described with emphasis on the extent and diversity of its associated problems. Mental health care represents a continuum from primary care to highly specialized services. The multi-faceted nature of mental illness and the range of services available to provide help, care and treatment are used to explore the roles and responsibilities of mental health nurses. The emphasis throughout the chapter will be on the values and principles which underpin good mental health practice. These include the involvement of **service users** and their carers, working in partnership, **social inclusion**, equality, teamwork and clinical effectiveness. The core of the chapter will discuss the attitudes, knowledge and skills required by mental health nurses, particularly in the development of an effective, **therapeutic** nurse–patient relationship and the delivery of **evidence-based interventions**. The educational pathway and preparation will be discussed in relation to the acquisition of skills and knowledge for mental health nursing training and the need for continuing education and life-long learning. The chapter will conclude by highlighting future trends, recent policy initiatives, advances in treatment and legislative reform, all of which impact on the future of mental health nursing.

SCENE SETTING

Achievements within mental health nursing

The past 50 years have seen enormous changes for mental health nurses both in their clinical practice and the way they are prepared for their role. Fifty years ago there was little effective treatment. People with a mental illness were sent to large asylums. At the time physical treatments predominated and mental health nurses were required to have medical and surgical skills to assist with insulin shock treatment, **psychosurgery** and **electroconvulsive** therapy. The 1960s brought in the widespread use of pharmaceutical interventions and a substantial increase in the understanding and management of mental illness. The resulting provision of community care and the closure of psychiatric hospitals provided mental health nurses with many opportunities and challenges. Despite the sometimes harmful and unwanted side-effects of prescribed medications there is no denying that they have relieved and reduced some of the major symptoms and distress associated with mental illness, including hallucinations and **delusions**. Pharmaceutical interventions have also enabled a much more multi-dimensional approach to treatments, such as group therapy, psychosocial interventions, cognitive behavioural therapy and family interventions. These positive advances together with a movement towards a more comprehensive range of care settings have enabled mental health nurses to respond to the needs of people with mental health problems with a range of evidence-based interventions that they can apply in a variety of service settings including primary care, acute inpatient care and highly specialized psychiatric units.

THE EXTENT AND INCIDENCE OF · MENTAL ILLNESS

In the UK, mental health is one of the government's four priority areas for the modernization programme of the National Health Service (NHS) with one adult in six (13 million people) experiencing one or other form of mental illness (Department of Health (DoH), 1999a). Mental health consumes 9 per cent of the NHS budget. In addition mental illness accounts for £32 billion of the health economy per year with £12 billion attributed to lost employment and £8 billion in benefits payments. Just as there are many different types of physical illness, mental illness is also multi-faceted. Mental illnesses range from the more common conditions such as depression to the more complex complaints such as schizophrenia. Unfortunately,

due to a number of reasons, mental illness does not receive the profile it deserves. This often results in misunderstanding, stigma and variation in services. People with mental illness are often socially excluded, have reduced opportunities for education and employment and a lack of supportive networks.

As part of its modernization programme the government is set to reverse this trend and launched a strategy and way forward for modern mental health services (DoH, 1998). The vision is to provide safe, sound and supportive services for patients and users. Among the proposals is a requirement for the NHS and social services to work together to provide a seamless and integrated service. Mental health has been given a much higher priority by the government with its inclusion among its programmes of National Service Frameworks (NSFs). The National Service Framework for Mental Health (Box 6.1) lays down models of treatment and care that people can expect wherever they live. It spells out national standards for mental health, which are founded on sound available evidence, what is achievable, how they should be developed and delivered and the ways performance will be measured in every part of the country.

Box 6.1 The National Service Framework Standards

Standard One

Health and social services should:

- promote mental health for all, working with individuals and communities
- combat discrimination against individuals and groups with mental health problems and promote their social inclusion

Standard Two

Any service user who contacts their primary care team with a common mental health problem should:

- have their mental health needs identified and assessed
- be offered effective treatments, including referral to specialist services for further assessment, treatment and care if they require it

Standard Three

Any individual with a common mental health problem should:

- be able to make contact round the clock with local services necessary to meet their needs and receive adequate care

- be able to use NHS Direct, as it develops, for first-level advice and referral on to specialist helplines or to local services

Standard Four

All mental health service users on the Care Programme Approach (CPA) should:

- receive care which optimizes engagement, prevents or anticipates crisis, and reduces risk
- have a copy of a written care plan which (i) includes the action to be taken in a crisis by service users, their carers, and their care co-ordinators, (ii) advises the general practitioner how they should respond if the service user needs additional help and (iii) is regularly reviewed by the care co-ordinator
- be able to access services 24 hours a day, 365 days a year

Standard Five

Each service user who is assessed as requiring a period of care away from their home should have:

- timely access to an appropriate hospital bed or alternative bed or place, which is (i) in the least restrictive environment consistent with the need to protect them and the public and (ii) as close to home as possible
- a copy of a written after care plan agreed on discharge, which sets out the care and rehabilitation to be provided, identifies the care co-ordinator, and specifies the action to be taken in a crisis

Standard Six

All individuals who provide regular and substantial care for a person on CPA should:

- have an assessment of their caring, physical and mental health needs, repeated on at least an annual basis
- have their own written care plan, which is given to them and implemented in discussion with them

Standard Seven

Local health and social care communities should prevent suicides by:

- promoting mental health for all, working with individuals and communities (Standard One)
- delivering high quality primary mental health care (Standard Two)
- ensuring that anyone with a mental health problem can contact local services via an accident and emergency department (Standard Three)
- ensuring that individuals with severe and enduring mental illness have a care plan which meets their specific needs, including access to services round the clock (Standard Four)
- providing safe hospital accommodation for individuals who need it (Standard Five)
- enabling individuals caring for someone with severe mental illness to receive the support which they need to continue to care (Standard Six)

and

- supporting local prison staff in preventing suicides among prisoners
- ensuring that staff are competent to assess the risk of suicide among individuals at greatest risk
- developing local systems for suicide audit to learn lessons and take any necessary action

Source: Department of Health (1999b)

The government acknowledges that implementation of the standards specified in the NSF will require additional staff, including nurses who are trained and supported. To ensure the creation of such a workforce the government has developed an action plan to address the following:

- workforce planning
- education and training
- recruitment and retention
- developing and supporting leadership.

In addition the action team provides national leadership in developing and taking forward the workforce plan. Following an assessment of the workforce implications of the NSF the Workforce Action Team proposed a mixture of practical, short-term initiatives to support the NSF and longer-term, more radical thinking which are meant to challenge some of the ways in which mental health workforce issues have been addressed previously. Included in the recommendations is the expectation that every region will map current education and training provision against the core competencies required to deliver the NSF (Brooker *et al.*, 2000). The Workforce Action Team also recommends the exploration of recruiting more professionally non-affiliated people and providing them with appropriate training. For example graduate mental health workers, support time recovery workers and gateway workers.

In parallel with these developments the DoH commissioned the Sainsbury Centre of Mental Health to establish a single agreed set of the competencies required to deliver each of the NSF standards. In October 2000 the Sainsbury Centre for Mental Health produced the Capability Framework and the list of practitioner capabilities required to implement the NSF. The report defines 'capability' by the following dimensions:

- a performance component which identifies what people need to possess and what they need to achieve in the workplace
- an ethical component that is concerned with integrating a knowledge of culture, values and social awareness into professional practice
- a component that emphasizes reflective practice

- the ability to effectively implement evidence-based interventions in the service configurations of a modern mental health system
- a commitment to working with new models of professional practice and responsibility for life-long learning.

The capabilities in the new framework are not specific to any profession and combine the notions of the effective practitioner with that of the reflective practitioner. The Capability Framework consists of values, attitudes and knowledge in addition to competencies along with an ability to apply these in practice across a range of clinical contexts. The Framework for Capable Practice produced by the Sainsbury Centre for Mental Health is shown in Appendix 4 on page 147.

Mental health nursing has often been threatened by the ambiguity expressed over the role of the mental health nurse in the multi-disciplinary setting and the calls for more blurring of professional roles. The recommendations for core competencies for all mental health staff and the suggestion for more professionally non-affiliated people to work in mental health may also be seen as a threat to the professional status of mental health nurses. Before exploring why the mental health nurses are essential members of the multi-disciplinary team it is worth reiterating one of the main findings of the Sainsbury report *Pulling Together: the future roles and training of mental health staff* (1997):

> the review found little evidence or support for radical reconfigurations of current professional boundaries. There is great value in diversity and each of the current mental health professions has strengths and skills to offer for the services of the future.

Why do we need mental health nurses?

'Making a difference' how mental health nurses are different and why they need to be

Fifty years ago the General Nursing Council (GNC) syllabus (GNC, 1957) reflected the belief that psychiatric nursing was very similar to general nursing (Thomas, 1992). A number of reports since have examined the roles and functions of mental health nurses. In 1968 a major review by the Ministry of Health highlighted the importance of counselling and psychotherapeutic skills. The report recognized that mental health nurses were required to play a much more active therapeutic role and should be prepared accordingly. In addition to preparing nurses for advanced clinical roles, such as psychological treatments including behaviour therapy, the importance of the therapeutic relationship was recognized. The therapeutic relationship is seen as central to effective care and much research has been carried out to identify the components of forming a good working relationship and its helpful, beneficial elements (Altschul, 1972; Cormack, 1983).

Despite the potential for mental health nurses to expand their therapeutic role, progress in general was slow, particularly on acute wards and recently the nature of the nursing work has begun reverting back to a custodial role. The introduction of the theory-orientated Project 2000 (UKCC, 2000) curriculum with its 18-month common foundation programme (CFP) also left many mental health nurses feeling inadequately prepared for their roles and lacking in practical skills. It was against this background that another ministerial review of mental health nursing took place. The review team, under the chairmanship of Professor Butterworth, were asked to 'Identify the future requirements for skilled nursing care in the light of developments in the provision of services for people with mental illness'.

The **Mental Health Nursing Review Team's report** (DoH, 1994) concluded that mental health nurses should focus on people with serious and enduring mental illness. In addition when addressing the individual needs of patients wherever possible the patient or service user should be fully involved in the care process including the development of care plans. The report clearly identified the core skills of mental health nurses but remained critical of the lack of post-registration courses and expressed concern over recruitment to mental health nursing. *Working in Partnership* (DoH, 1994) captured the essence and the principles underlying user involvement and user empowerment. The report recommended that:

Mental health nursing should re-examine every aspect of its policy and practice in the light of

the needs of the people who use services. Nursing services should be designed and developed to meet the needs of service users and people should not be expected to conform to the convenience of the service.

Working in Partnership set a major challenge for mental health nurses. It questioned accepted practice and enabled mental health nurses to become the forerunners at facilitating user involvement and treating people who use mental health services more as equal partners rather than passive recipients. Most recently, the *Chief Nursing Officer's Review of Mental Health Nursing*, due to be published early in 2006, is likely to include changes and improvements for pre-registration training provided in both academic and practice settings (DoH, 2005).

Users' rights and user involvement

The mental health service user movement has a long history, however, it is only since the mid-1980s that the cause has gained momentum in the UK. Since that time many improvements brought about in mental health services have occurred because of listening to and working with the people who use the services. The first of 10 guiding values and principles underpinning the National Service Framework for Mental Health (DoH, 1999b) clearly identifies the expectation that services will involve service users and their carers in the planning and delivery of care. A range of models have developed all seeking to integrate more genuine participation of service users and carers. These include patient satisfaction surveys, newsletters, user and carer support groups, advocacy projects, patients' councils and user-focused monitoring of services (Rose *et al.*, 1998).

It has been suggested that on occasions mental health nurses will act as advocates for patients to empower them to make informed choices. Acting as the patient's advocate is often claimed as an integral part of the mental health nurse's role. The Royal College of Nursing (RCN, 1991) defines advocacy as 'a process of acting for and on behalf of someone who is unable to function themselves'. The principle of advocacy has been included in the **International Council of Nurses' Code** since the early 1970s. The RCN included advocacy as a practice function in its document *The Nature and Scope of Professional Practice* (RCN, 1991). However despite official endorsements from international and national nursing bodies, advocacy in nursing has not been universally understood, accepted or adopted. The reasons for this are multi-faceted. In a review of the literature Mallik (1997) found that despite a considerable increase in the claims by nurses to undertake the patient advocacy role, in the past 20 years confusion still exists about the complexities and potential problems inherent in the role of advocate.

In describing the history of advocacy in mental health David and Toby Brandon (2000) raise the thorny issue of professionals acting as patient advocates. Although the nurse–patient relationship remains pivotal to mental health nursing, the advocacy role is increasingly undertaken by independent agencies. Currently a range of **advocacy agencies** exist well outside of conventional mental health services where independence is the fundamental principle. These advocates offer a range of services including advice, information giving, befriending, support and practical assistance. Although there is a new legitimacy and availability of advocacy services, Kerr (1997) suggests that the keys to successful advocacy are accountability, focus and support. He proposes that advocates must be answerable not only to their clients and potential clients, but also to their funders and the professionals with whom they work. Advocates must seek to engage with all parties on a basis of trust and co-operation according to Kerr. Finally he suggests that there is national need to evaluate advocacy services and for greater sharing and learning between projects.

The NHS Plan (DoH, 2000) emphasizes the importance of putting the patient at the centre of the NHS. The resulting publication of the **Health and Social Care Bill** (House of Commons, 2000) addresses these arrangements and covers the developments in the planning of a more robust system of patient and public involvement. The new arrangements offer a broader scope of involvement including:

- all NHS organizations have a statutory duty to consult and involve patients and the public
- there will be a patient's forum for each NHS trust and each primary care trust (PCT)

- patients' fora will be independent statutory bodies, whose primary function is the monitoring and review of health services from the patient's perspective.

WHAT CAN BE ACHIEVED THROUGH EFFECTIVE MENTAL HEALTH NURSING?

Evidence of value of mental health nursing

As well as putting the service user first, contemporary mental health nursing seeks to provide care in accordance with the best available evidence. Rather than nursing care being based upon traditional custom and practice, nurses are expected to know the available evidence which supports the interventions of their choice. The available evidence should also be integrated with individual clinical experience and service user choice (Geddes *et al.*, 1999). However, there are many mental health nursing interventions where information is imperfect and there is a shortage of evidence. Even when evidence is available, it is based on a small number of studies which often lack scientific rigour. Also there is the practical problem of accessing the necessary information. There are, however, a number of ways to access up-to-date good quality research findings and clinical guidelines. Generally, there are five main levels of evidence:

- randomized control trials
- systematic reviews
- non-randomized experimental studies
- non-experimental studies
- expert opinion.

Accepted methods of accessing such evidence include searching databases, journals and bulletins such as *Evidence-Based Mental Health* (see Useful websites at the end of this chapter).

Evidence-based practice

Like other professional groups mental health nurses have found it difficult to implement research findings into clinical practice (McKenna, 1995; Yonge *et al.*, 1997). However, more recently a number of research-validated interventions, although not widely disseminated, have become more estab-lished in nursing practice. These include psychoso-cial interventions which are normally divided into three main categories according to their general aims and clinical procedures (Tarrier *et al.*, 1998) These are:

- Family interventions
- Cognitive–behavioural therapy (CBT)
- Early sign monitoring and early interventions

Family interventions

Family interventions arose primarily from research on expressed emotion (EE). Rigorous studies have consistently shown that service users who returned home to live with relatives and who rated high on EE were much more likely to relapse than those who went back to live with relatives having low EE (Kavanagh, 1992). In the belief that changing the behaviour of relatives with high EE would reduce the risk of relapse, a number of interven-tions have been designed to lower stress in the home situation. Common features among these interventions includes an educational, information-giving aspect, a problem-solving approach and assisting the family to develop coping strategies. Tarrier *et al.* (1998) suggest that methodologically sound clinical research has consistently found that family intervention in conjunction with **prophy-lactic** medication reduces relapse rates in people with **schizophrenia**, at least in the short and medium term. However, despite these findings the numbers of mental health nurses who carry out family interventions remain low.

Cognitive–behavioural therapy for psychotic symptoms

Since the 1990s research is showing increasingly that psychotic and affective symptoms can be reduced using CBT. These interventions consist of a number of different treatments including prob-lem solving, coping strategy enhancement and management of auditory hallucinations. Although the results are encouraging most of the research so far has been single case design (Fowler *et al.*, 1995). Controlled trials will add to our body of knowledge about the effectiveness of CBT in the treatment of **psychotic** symptoms. Many mental health nurses have now been trained in CBT.

Early intervention

Early intervention in **psychosis** usually involves three main areas:

- services based in primary care
- intensive treatment at onset
- detection of **prodromal signs** in people prone to relapse.

Hirsch and Jolley (1989) found that 70 per cent of service users who relapsed complained of 'a fear of going crazy'. This led them to believe that service users can usually tell when they are becom-ing unwell but can not always articulate or define these feelings. Birchwood and Shepherd (1992) demonstrate that early intervention at the first signs of relapse including stress reduction and a review of medication are effective in preventing relapse. Mental health nurses have a key role to play helping service users and their carers identify and monitor these early signs and seek appropriate treatment sooner. For a fuller review of the latest evidence in these approaches see Wykes *et al.* (1998).

As previously mentioned a number of studies have examined the impact of psychosocial inter-vention training on routine nursing practice. Unfortunately implementation remains problem-atic for a number of reasons. These include out-dated teaching methods, organizational barriers, resistance to change and lack of clinically compe-tent supervisors.

The Report by the Standing Nursing and Midwifery Advisory Committee (SNMAC), (DoH, 1999c) suggests that in recent years the focus of education, training, status and career opportun-ities have all shifted from acute in-patient care to the community and specialist services. Despite the increasingly demanding nature of in-patient care it is not seen as an attractive area to work in and does not attract the required expertise. The SNMAC sub-committee found a number of skill deficits in mental health nurses working in acute in-patients including evidence-based cognitive, behavioural and family interventions.

Many of the new mental health nurse training programmes are addressing these deficits. For example the Thorn Programme aims to equip nurses with skills in a range of interventions to meet the needs of people with psychotic symp-toms and their families. Students are taught case management, CBT and family interventions.

Unfortunately, as previously mentioned good-quality evidence is not available in all areas and where it is lacking it is important to seek out established clinical principles, procedures, policies and guidelines from professional organizations, for example *Practice Guidance: safe and supportive observation of patients at risk* (SNMAC, 1999).

The drive for evidence-based care is long overdue. Most mental health nurses have been taught to avoid doing harm while trying to help people with mental health problems on the road to recovery. Unfortunately, even today few of the interventions used have been found by scientific research to be of established benefit. This paucity of knowledge is not just peculiar to mental health nursing but persists throughout the profession. While, at last, some headway has been made in the identification of useful interventions, for the foreseeable future, mental health nurses will continue to provide care without knowing if what we are doing is effective. The balance between potential benefit and risk has to be assessed in every situation.

Summary

The emphasis in mental health care is changing towards evidence-based practice. However, it is not enough for interventions to have proved therapeutic effectiveness. They must be acceptable to service users and be delivered sensitively, otherwise they will be regarded as ineffective. It is therefore important to gather evidence through the use of patient feedback. Service users can provide valuable feedback on the quality of care they receive. For example a number of studies have investigated what service users have found helpful about the care provided by mental health nurses (Beech and Norman, 1995; Cutcliffe and Bassett, 1997). This growing body of evidence suggests that service users find nursing interventions based in human relationships, including empathy, respect and dignity, and good communication skills most helpful.

CLINICAL GOVERNANCE, CLINICAL EFFECTIVENESS AND RISK MANAGEMENT

Clinical governance is the umbrella term for all those activities aimed at improving patient care. Some of these have already been described in the previous sections. In addition clinical governance involves clinical effectiveness; the setting, delivering and monitoring of standards; **clinical audit**; creating an open learning culture and sharing information. Clinical governance is underpinned by leadership, continuing professional development and professional self-regulation. All of these concepts are central to current health reforms.

> Clinical effectiveness is about doing the right thing in the right way for the right patient.
>
> (RCN, 1996)

In addition to making sure the care provided is based on sound research evidence and informed service user preference, clinical effectiveness involves a consistent approach. It is important that mental health nurses are able to think about and question their practice. To do so they need to work within a culture that encourages open and frank discussions; a culture where reflection and learning from experience is part of day-to-day practice. This includes acknowledging what is effective and works, learning from mistakes and what is ineffective. In order to encourage such learning, there must be a blame-free culture rather than one that is punitive and where standard practice is to take disciplinary action.

KNOWLEDGE AND SKILLS OF MENTAL HEALTH NURSES

Working in Partnership (DoH, 1994), the report of the mental health nursing review team, identified the skills of the mental health nurse in relation to the phases of the nursing process; assessment, planning, implementation and evaluation. A wide range of specific skills are identified under broad headings related to each phase. Box 6.2 provides a few examples from the whole range. It is these core skills, based on the therapeutic use of self in the nurse–patient relationship, in conjunction with a client-centred philosophy, values and practice that

Box 6.2 Working in Partnership: skills of the mental health nurse

Assessment

- Self-awareness, e.g. awareness of one's own degree of attention to others
- Observing, e.g. how others react to the individual
- Data collection, e.g. awareness of sources of data – individual, family and significant others including other professionals
- Interviewing, e.g. listening and attending
- Identifying needs and diagnosing problems, e.g. recognizing issues amenable to nursing intervention and identifying those which need to be referred to others
- Recording and disseminating information, e.g. organizing, documenting, charting, processing and assembling information

Planning

- Identifying solutions, e.g. using problem-solving skills to generate creative solutions
- Setting goals, e.g. setting short-term and long-term objectives of nursing care, taking account of the policies of the organization
- Formulating plans, e.g. setting the criteria of evaluation for measuring the achievement of objectives
- Communicating, e.g. negotiating the care plan with the individual and the care team
- Producing the plan, e.g. writing a clearly expressed unique nursing care plan which can be understood by all grades of the multi-disciplinary team

Implementation

- Planned intervention, e.g. modifying objectives in the light of further information
- Motivating, e.g. using positive incentives, persuasion, suggestion, appropriate rewards
- Teaching, e.g. identifying and agreeing learning needs
- Managing, e.g. maintaining a positive attitude
- Meeting personal care needs, e.g. promotion of independence
- Organization, e.g. effective organization of the environment

Evaluation

- Defining results, e.g. identifying methods of evaluation
- Obtaining feedback, e.g. discriminating between what is valid and invalid
- Assessing results, e.g. assessing the validity and reliability of data of the evaluation
- Identifying process changes required, e.g. using the results of evaluation to reconsider nursing care plans
- Creating opportunities, e.g. identifying realistic short- and long-term goals for change
- Reviewing overall performance, e.g. reviewing with the team the results achieved
- Managing success/failure in achieving goals, e.g. identifying what was effective and ineffective within the constraints
- Recording and communicating, e.g. documenting the progress achieved against criteria

Source: DoH (1994)

is responsive to individual need that provides the unique experience of mental health nursing.

While it is important to identify and articulate clearly core skills, values and knowledge – the unique contribution of mental health nursing – it is important to see the relationships between these attributes and those that are common to the nursing profession as a whole and to other professional and occupational groups. The Sainsbury Centre for Mental Health has addressed the future roles and training of mental health staff. *Pulling Together* (1997) identifies the skills, knowledge and attitudes required in mental health services across different professional groups. The report sets out core competencies for working with adults with severe mental illness (Box 6.3) as the basis for a training framework providing 'fitness for purpose' of staff working with people with severe mental illness. The unique and various skills of the different disciplines may be built around such a framework.

Box 6.3 Core skills, knowledge and attitudes for mental health workers

Management and administration

- Knowledge of current systems of care and the policy background (CPA, supervision registers, community care and care management procedures, functions and organization of primary care)
- Understanding of mental health law and related legislation, especially in relation to users' civil rights and powers of compulsion and detention
- Understanding the roles of the various disciplines and agencies involved in the provision of mental health care and the range of settings within which care and treatment take place
- Awareness of the role and contribution of non-specialist and support staff, and the ability to supervise and provide support to those staff

Assessment

- Skill in conducting a collaborative needs-based assessment
- Ability to develop a treatment and care plan based on a thorough and comprehensive assessment of the client, family and social system
- Apply knowledge of the issues and skill in the assessment and management of the combined problem of drug and alcohol abuse and mental illness
- Skills in the assessment of users' needs and requirements of housing, occupation and income
- Apply knowledge and skill in risk assessment and the management of violence and aggression
- Apply knowledge of factors related to the development of 'chronic crises' and skill in assessment and management strategies

Treatment and care management

- Knowledge of the priority target group, their needs, characteristics and clinical symptomatology
- Knowledge of crisis intervention, theory and practice
- Effective understanding of current medical interventions and possible side-effects
- Knowledge of basic current cognitive–behavioural strategies to assist users, carers and family networks to contain and manage a severe and enduring mental illness
- Understanding of the issues in the evaluation and treatment of service users at risk of self-harm or suicidal behaviour
- Knowledge and skill in effective interpersonal communication
- Awareness of cultural and gender issues in mental illness and an awareness of the principles and practices of anti-discriminatory and anti-racist practice

- Knowledge and skill in creating therapeutic co-operation and developing an alliance with the service user
- Awareness of the needs, characteristics and principles of care for homeless people with mental illness
- Knowledge and skill in the provision of assertive outreach and long-term continuing care
- Awareness of the needs, characteristics and principles of care for forensic patients
- Awareness of user perspectives on the provision of treatment and continuing care
- Knowledge of care management principles

Collaborative working

- Awareness of the need to work in partnership with carers and social networks
- Ability to work effectively as a member of a multi-disciplinary mental health team through clarity about the role and purpose of the team and its individual members
- Understanding of sources of conflict and development of basic teamwork skills including negotiation and conflict resolution
- Comprehension of the need for and willingness to participate effectively in multi-disciplinary teams

Source: Sainsbury Centre for Mental Health (1997)

The United Kingdom Central Council for Nursing Midwifery and Health Visiting (NMC, 2004; DoH 2001, 2004) have identified four domains common to all areas of nursing along with competencies required for entry to the register. These competencies – common to all areas of nursing – are the starting point of a career in nursing (see also Appendix 2). Specific competencies or benchmarks for mental health nursing to be achieved on completion of the mental health branch programme have also been identified and cross referenced with the UKCC competencies and domains (The Northern Centre for Mental Health and The Northern and Yorkshire Regional Education and Workforce Development Subgroup for Mental Health, 2000). This marks a new development in the pre-registration programme for preparation and registration as a mental health nurse. The next section addresses nurse training and education.

MENTAL HEALTH NURSING EDUCATION AND TRAINING

The ENB (2000) and the UKCC (1999) identify broad guiding principles that underpin requirements for programmes leading to registration on the professional register as a qualified nurse. These guiding principles are related to competencies and outcomes that need to be achieved during the period of training and preparation and provide the foundation for outcome-based competencies.

In September 2000 a new model of training started in 16 university pilot sites across the UK. This new outcomes competency-based model had its roots in the government's White Paper *Making A Difference* (DoH, 1999d). This called for a common approach to definition of outcomes for programmes leading to registration to ensure that newly qualified nurses and midwives are fit to practise.

A Commission for Education was established by the UKCC in 1999 to address plans to improve nurse education and training. Priorities included:

- more flexible career pathways into and within nursing and midwifery education
- develop a training system that is more responsive to the modern NHS
- stronger practical orientation to pre-registration training.

Fitness for Practice, the report of the Commission for Education (UKCC, 1999) (also referred to as The Peach Report after Sir Leonard

Peach, Chair of the Commission) reviewed evaluations of Project 2000, established in the 1980s as the means of preparing nurses and midwives, identifying its achievements and deficits. Identifying key drivers for change, the report of the Commission established a new approach to training, building and maintaining a workforce for the NHS. This new model of health-needs-led education would focus on:

- the contemporary and anticipated needs of health care
- an outcome-based competency approach to fitness for practice
- sound assessment of practice and its integration with theory.

This new approach would provide:

- A consistent, standardized approach to nurse education
- Wider access to nurse training
- Strengthening links between vocational training and pre-registration education
- Vocational pathways into nurse training
- More part-time training opportunities
- Fast-track nurse training
- Recognition of life experiences as preparation to be a carer
- Students to feel part of the NHS
- NHS employers recognize their obligation to students.

OUTCOMES-BASED COMPETENCE FOR NURSE EDUCATION

Common Foundation Programme

A 1-year CFP prepares students to a common level of competence for entry into the branch programme. Standards for entry to the CFP and the branch programmes have become more flexible. National Vocational Qualifications (NVQs), access programmes, Accreditation of Prior Learning (APL) and Accreditation of Prior (Experiential) Learning (AP(E)L) are increasingly recognized for entry into nurse training. Both diploma and degree-level pathways to mental health nursing are available.

Widening access and flexibility may be more attractive to health care assistants, nurse cadets and support workers necessary for the workforce of the modern health service. Training should allow breaks in studies at specified points – allowing you to work in the health service – with recognition and reward for your achievement and experience to date. Those students who wish to leave the training programme at the end of year 1/CFP will be awarded both academic and practice credit according to their experience relating to the appropriate credit framework, e.g. credits towards NVQs/SVQs.

During year 1, the CFP and throughout the branch programme students are introduced to and experience a range of different approaches to teaching and learning. While this involves the provision and acquisition of information and knowledge through lectures and tutorials, an increasing amount of training and education involves more learner-centred approaches. The emphasis of these approaches is on output and outcomes – the identification and provision of evidence to validate competence.

Being competent involves more than being able to demonstrate an ability to carry out certain tasks. Competence is defined in *Fit for Practice* as 'the skills and ability to practise safely and effectively without direct supervision' (UKCC, 1999). The increased emphasis on practise-based learning highlights the importance of learning that takes place in the practice setting as an important part of the academic award.

Outcomes-based education is student-centred and facilitative – an approach which acknowledges that learning takes place in a practice setting is as valuable as that taking place in an academic institution. Outcome-based standards address competence in both theory and practice. In the CFP there is early emphasis on practice skills and learning from clinical experience gained in clinical placements. Learning outcomes are achieved through the development of knowledge and understanding facilitated through group work and work-based learning. Experiential and problem-based learning skills laboratories and information technology are educational approaches that may be used to facilitate learning during practice placements.

Educational progression is monitored through the use of evidence-based practice portfolios, self-assessment and reflective accounts of learning from clinical experience. These portfolios are used to provide evidence of rational decision-making and clinical judgement demonstrating a student's fitness for practice. During periods of clinical experience your practice will be assessed by a trained assessor against specific performance criteria relevant to the stage of the programme. The practice portfolio is used to keep a record of observations related to these performance criteria. These count as evidence, measures of progress and experience toward the outcomes of the programme.

What is the mental health branch?

The mental health branch, normally two years in duration, is the route to professional registration as a mental health nurse. Mental health nurses use the relationship they develop with an individual who has mental health problems to help them come to terms with, gain an understanding of and cope with their experience. To achieve this students undertaking the mental health branch need a sound understanding of social interaction and social relationships, positive and negative effects of responding to and managing stress, crisis and change among individuals and groups. They also need to know what they bring to their relationships with others, an awareness of their own personal attributes and characteristics and the effect of these on their relationships with others.

This may seem a tall order to achieve in a lifetime let alone a 2-year branch programme. However, these attitudes and values are central to mental health nursing and are developed through the branch programme. Like most occupations and professions, mental health nursing has its own share of stereotypes and clichés – some negative, some positive – for example:

- 'They just sit around drinking cups of tea'
- 'Laid back'
- 'Wanting to psychoanalyse everybody'
- 'In it to sort themselves out'
- 'Able to "simply" be with someone when they are distressed and having a bad time – it actually takes great personal strength'
- 'Totally non-judgemental'
- 'Well-grounded individuals'
- 'Treating each individual as unique'

- 'They are really good listeners – they engage and involve people who would otherwise be excluded'
- 'They see the whole picture – where the individual is on their own life journey'.

An interest in and sense of the way people relate to each other, how they feel about themselves and about others, developing and using self-awareness, self-confidence and self-esteem in everyday interactions are important qualities that can be further developed as a mental health nurse. The ability to be with someone, simply and calmly, for them, while they are acutely distressed – rather than try to make things better, explain why, or change the subject – things most people do to make *themselves* feel more comfortable about someone else's distress – is an important quality among nurses and carers, but particularly so among mental health nurses. The expression 'Don't just do something – sit there!' is rather apt.

Supervised practice and preceptorship

Towards the end of the mental health branch all students undertake a period of supervised clinical practice where they consolidate their education and competence in practice. This period, normally at least 3 months in duration, is a transitional period with clearly specified role-related outcomes that is managed by a specifically prepared registered nurse.

Following registration, and on commencement of employment as a mental health nurse all newly qualified practitioners undergo a period of preceptorship. This involves a planned and organized induction programme with the support they will need to assume the role and responsibilities of a qualified practitioner who is accountable for his or her own clinical practice.

CLINICAL EXPERIENCE

The outcomes-based competency curriculum marks the most recent change in the preparation and training of nurses, a change that shifts the emphasis onto the clinical practice setting for the development of the necessary skills, knowledge and understanding. Currently student nurses are expected to spend 50 per cent of their training in clinical placements.

In the past, the quality of the learning environment and practice experiences have varied considerably from one placement to the next. One of the main aims of the outcomes-based competency curriculum is to improve the overall quality of learning from clinical experience. This involves longer placements and initiatives that make clinical placements a better, more supportive learning environment for the student. These include increased teacher support for students on placement and increasing the number of staff involved in supporting students who have joint appointments between universities, NHS trusts, social care and other service organizations, for example lecturer practitioners and practice educators.

Longer practice placements allow students to develop a range of skills, including interpersonal skills with individuals experiencing mental health problems and working with groups of clients over a period of time. Longer placements will also allow students to experience how the organization of nursing work, i.e. day and night shifts covering 24-hour periods seven days a week, out-reach, liaison and consultation impact on the care of clients in different settings. They will gain a better understanding of working practices in the health care environment.

Placements should reflect service delivery and are likely to involve services for the elderly mentally ill, acute in-patient units, community services and community mental health teams. The development of mental health promotion strategies in line with the NSF for mental health emphasize liaison and consultation with primary care services and general practices and will provide new types of clinical experience and different opportunities for a range of practice experiences. Some placements may be with new and developing services such as general hospital accident and emergency departments providing liaison psychiatric nursing services for people who self-harm. They may also involve user groups, rehabilitation and employment-focused services and support, services for children with mental health problems, family work, people with dependency problems associated with the use of drugs and alcohol.

THE NEXT STEPS

Life-long learning and continuous professional development

As highlighted in the section on clinical governance there is a clear expectation that mental health nurses will be committed to continuing professional development (CPD) and life-long learning. Ideally every nurse should have a personal development plan linked to performance appraisal and organizational objectives. The government's strategic intentions for nurses outlined in *Making a Difference* (DoH, 1999d) suggests that in planning or providing CPD organizations should ensure that it contains the requirements listed in Table 5 of the document (p. 29). Continuing professional development, complemented by a knowledge and skills framework is key to the government's proposals for a new pay system *Agenda for Change* (DoH, 1999a).

In addition to meeting the personal and professional development needs of nurses CPD programmes need to meet local service needs. As local services set about implementing the standards contained in the NSF much of their successful delivery will depend on the skills and ability of mental health nurses. There are enormous opportunities for nurses to work with a range of disciplines and contribute to these new developments. These developments include:

- assertive out-reach
- early intervention in psychosis
- mental health promotion strategies
- strengthening primary mental health care
- accident and emergency mental health liaison services
- crisis resolution, home treatment and crisis management.

Specialist practice

Mental health nurses work in a variety of settings and with a range of specific service user groups. Many of these have become highly specialized areas of practice and have their own particular post-registration training. These include:

- Substance misuse
- Forensic mental health nursing

- Child and adolescent mental health
- Eating disorders
- Older people and mental health.

A full description of the services available for these particular groups and the latest approaches to their nursing care is beyond the scope of this chapter. For a concise educational tour of specialist mental health nursing see *Stuart and Sundeen's Mental Health Nursing: Principles and practice* (Thomas *et al.*, 1997).

SUMMARY AND CONCLUSIONS
A vision for the future

So what of the future of mental health nursing? We know that mental illness is likely to increase and that there will be greater numbers of mentally disordered offenders. To address these increases the UK government has produced a range of key underpinning programmes and an investment of an extra £700 million over the next 3 years in mental health services. This will fund an increase in the number of medium secure beds, more outreach services including crisis teams and 24-hour care. All of these modern services call for an increase both in the numbers, knowledge and skills of mental health nurses.

Occupational standards, capabilities and competencies

The outcomes-based competency curriculum, developed through nursing programmes in higher education institutions, draws together occupational and academic standards in a new approach to professional preparation. This together with the government's 10-year strategy for reforming mental health services with an emphasis on multi-agency and multi-disciplinary working, with partnerships between health and social care sets the future agenda.

It appears that the various approaches to identifying core attributes and characteristics of mental health workers, for example the skills of the mental health nurse identified in *Working in Partnership* and the core competencies identified in *Pulling Together*, will be consolidated in terms of the way they relate to both criteria for professional and national occupational standards. Mapping generic competencies and capabilities for mental health work against the outcomes for the mental health branch programme for nurses and, similarly, the preparation of other professional groups will lead to a standardization of training and educational preparation of individuals working in this field. The identification of core and specific characteristics among mental health professionals will impact upon traditional boundaries of professional roles and professional identity. This will clarify the specific contribution of different professional and occupational groups and increase awareness of the importance of collaborative multi-disciplinary teamwork.

The Department of Health is also supporting the development of national occupational standards for mental health. Healthwork UK, the health care national training organization has set out key areas and key roles for those involved in providing mental health care. Each of the key areas identified in the list below is associated with key roles and functions.

1 Work in partnership with individuals, groups and agencies to promote mental health and combat discrimination against those with mental health needs.
2 Assess mental health needs, diagnose mental illness, plan, implement and review programmes of treatment and care in the broader context of individual lives.
3 Plan, provide, implement and review interventions to address the individual's mental health needs and provide ongoing support, rehabilitation and continuing care.
4 Develop and maintain safe, stimulating and secure environments for individuals who have mental health needs.
5 Manage the risk to the public of offending behaviour by individuals with mental health needs and develop, implement and review programmes and interventions to address individuals' offending behaviour.
6 Develop, maintain and improve ethical, evidence-based practice which promotes communication and relationships with individuals, their careers and other agencies.

7 Develop strategies, policies and services for improving mental health and addressing mental illness, and manage people, resources and information.

Mental health nurses have a major role to play in each of these key areas. The chapter has highlighted the numerous initiatives aimed at achieving a workforce that is fit for the purpose of delivering a modern mental health service. These initiatives together with new service configurations and developments have major implications for the education and training of mental health nurses. There has never been a more exciting time to undertake mental health nurse training. For the first time there is an opportunity to have a system of education and training reflecting service need and workforce requirements that have a growing evidence base; all of which will be underpinned by the views of service users, those who support them, and provide them with more purposeful nursing care and a mental health service that meets their needs and expectations.

GLOSSARY

In the context of this chapter the meanings of the following words are described:

Advocacy agencies	Organizations or groups that provide support to or campaign on behalf of people with mental health problems
Clinical audit	Comparison of existing clinical practice against agreed professional standards based on reliable evidence and patient outcomes
Delusion	False belief strongly held in spite of invalidating evidence, especially as a symptom of mental illness, e.g. delusions of persecution
Electroconvulsive therapy (ECT)	Administration of electric current to the brain through electrodes placed on the head, usually near the temples to induce unconsciousness and brief convulsions. Used in the treatment of certain mental disorders, especially acute depression
Evidence-based interventions	Actions that aim to improve the health and well-being of individuals, families and populations planned and delivered with due weight accorded to all valid, relevant information
Prodromal	Early or premonitory symptom of a disease
Prophylactic	Acting to defend against or prevent something, especially disease, e.g. protective drug or vaccine
Psychosurgery	Brain surgery used to treat severe, intractable mental or behavioural disorders
Psychosis	Severe mental disorder, with or without organic damage, characterized by derangement of personality and loss of contact with reality and causing deterioration of normal social functioning
Psychotic	Of, relating to or affected by psychosis
Schizophrenia	Psychotic disorder characterized by loss of contact with the environment, withdrawal from reality with noticeable deterioration in the level of functioning in everyday life, and by disintegration of personality expressed as disorder of feeling, thought (as in hallucinations and delusions), and conduct
Service users	People with mental health problems or mental illness who use mental health services
Social inclusion	Achieved when individuals or populations do not suffer from the negative aspects of unemployment, poor skills, low income, poor housing, crime, bad health, family problems, limited access to services and rurality, e.g. remoteness, sparsity, isolation and high costs
Therapeutic	Having or exhibiting healing properties

REFERENCES

Altschul AT (1972) *Nurse–patient Interaction: a study of interaction patterns in acute psychiatric wards.* Edinburgh: Churchill Livingstone.

Beech P, Norman I (1995) Patents' perceptions of quality of psychiatric nursing care: findings from a small scale descriptive study. *Journal of Clinical Nursing* 4: 117–23.

Birchwood M, Shepherd G (1992) Controversies and growing points in cognitive-behavioural interventions for people with schizophrenias. *Behavioural Psychotherapy* 20: 305–42.

Brandon D, Brandon T (2000) The history of advocacy in mental health. *Mental Health Practice* 3:6–8.

Brooker C, Gournay K, O'Halloran P, Bailey D (2000) Mapping training to support the implementation of the national service framework for Mental Health. ScHarr: University of Sheffield, Sheffield.

Cormack D (1983) *Psychiatric Nursing Described.* Edinburgh: Churchill Livingstone.

Cutcliffe J, Bassett C (1997) Introducing change in nursing: the case of research. *Journal of Nursing Management* 5: 241–7.

Department of Health (1994) *Working in Partnership: A collaborative approach to care.* London: DoH.

Department of Health (1998) *Modernising Mental Health Services.* London: DoH.

Department of Health (1999a) *Agenda for Change: modernising the NHS pay system.* London: DoH.

Department of Health (1999b) *The National Service Framework for Mental Health: Modern standards and service models.* London: DoH.

Department of Health (1999c) *Mental Health Nursing: Addressing acute concerns. Report by the Standing Nursing and Midwifery Advisory Committee.* London: DoH.

Department of Health (1999d) *Making a Difference. Strengthening the nursing, midwifery and health visiting contribution to health and health care.* London: DoH.

Department of Health (2000) *The NHS Plan: a plan for investment, a plan for reform.* London: DoH.

Department of Health (2001) Chief Executive Bulletin, Issue 94, 23–29 November, National Occupational Standards in Mental Health.

Department of Health (2004) *The Ten Essential Shared Capabilities – a framework for the whole of the mental health workforce.* London: DoH.

Department of Health (2005) *Chief Nursing Officer's Review of Mental Health Nursing.* London: DoH.

Fowler D, Garety PA, Kuipers L (1995) *Cognitive Behaviour Therapy for People with Psychosis.* Chichester: John Wiley and Sons.

Geddes J, Tomlin A, Price J (1999) *Practising Evidence-based Mental Health.* Oxford: Radcliffe Medical Press.

General Nursing Council (1957) *Guide to the Training Scheme for Nurses for Mental Diseases.* London: General Nursing Council for England and Wales.

Hirsch S, Jolley A (1989) The dysphoric syndrome in schizophrenia and its implications for relapse. *British Journal of Psychiatry* (suppl 5):46–50.

House of Commons (2000) Health and Social Care Bill (*Bill 9*). London: HMSO.

Kavanagh D (1992) Recent developments in expressed emotion and schizophrenia. *British Journal of Psychiatry* 160:601–20.

Kerr G (1997) Advocating advocacy. *Open Mind* 84:12.

Mallik M (1997) Advocacy in nursing: perceptions and attitudes of the nursing elite in the United Kingdom. *Journal of Advanced Nursing* 28:1001–11.

McKenna HP (1995) Dissemination and application of mental health. *Nursing Research* 4:1257–63.

Ministry of Health (1968) *Psychiatric Nursing Today and Tomorrow.* London: Mental Health Nursing Advisory Committee.

Northern Centre for Mental Health and the Northern and Yorkshire Regional Education and Workforce Development sub-group for mental health (2000) *A Competence-Based 'Exit Profile' for Pre-Registration Mental Health Nursing.* Durham: Northern Centre for Mental Health.

Rose D, Ford R, Lindley P, Gawith G and the KCW Mental Health Monitoring Users' Group (1998) *In Our Experience: User-focused monitoring of mental health services in Kensington and Chelsea and Westminster Health Authority.* London: Sainsbury Centre for Mental Health.

Royal College of Nursing (1991) *The Nature and Scope of Professional Practice.* London: RCN.

Royal College of Nursing (1996) *Doing the Right Thing: Clinical effectiveness for nurses.* London: RCN.

Sainsbury Centre for Mental Health (2000) *The Capable Practitioner: A framework and list of the practitioner capabilities required to implement the National Service Framework for Mental Health.* London: Sainsbury Centre for Mental Health.

Sainsbury Centre for Mental Health (1997) *Pulling Together: the future roles and training of mental health staff.* London: Sainsbury Centre for Mental Health.

Standing Nursing and Midwifery Advisory Committee (1999) *Practice Guidance: safe and supportive observation of patients at risk.* London: DoH.

Tarrier N, Hadock G, Barrowclough C (1998) Training and dissemination: research to practice in innovative psychological treatments for schizophrenia. In: Wylkes T, Tarrier N, Lewis S (eds) *Outcome and Innovation in Psychological Treatment of Schizophrenia.* Chichester: John Wiley & Sons.

Thomas B (1992) Education. In: Brooking J, Ritter S, Thomas B (eds) *A Textbook for Psychiatric and Mental Health Nursing.* Edinburgh: Churchill Livingstone.

Thomas B, Hardy S, Cutting P (1997) *Stuart and Sundeen's Principles and Practice of Mental Health Nursing.* Edinburgh: Mosby-Wolfe.

UKCC (1986) *Project 2000: A new preparation for practice.* London: UKCC.

United Kingdom Central Council for Nursing, Midwifery and Health Visiting (1999) *Fitness for Practice: The UKCC Commission for Nursing and Midwifery Education.* London: UKCC.

Wykes T, Tarrier N, Lewis S (1998) *Outcome and Innovation in Psychological Treatment of Schzophrenia.* Chichester: John Wiley & Sons.

Yonge I, Austin W, Zhou Qiuping P et al. (1997) A systematic review of the psychiatric/mental health nursing research literature 1982–1992. *Journal of Psychiatric Mental Health Nursing* 4:171–7.

ANNOTATED FURTHER READING

Thomson T, Mathias P (eds) (2003) *Lyttle's Mental Health and Disorder*, 3rd edn. London: Bailliere Tindall, RCN. This is a useful textbook for mental health nursing students including a broad range of contents under four main headings – Understanding mental health and illness, Interventions in mental health practice, Challenges for service delivery and Issues for practitioners. These four sections include a range of relevant topics, the nature of mental health, language and classification, emotion, behaviour and cognition, interventions including mental health promotion, social and psychological interventions, social inclusion, suicide and self-harm, substance use, and aggression management. The final section includes chapters on the development of high standards, supporting practitioners as they develop their knowledge and skills. The book includes a glossary of common mental health terms that students may find helpful.

Thomas B, Hardy S, Cutting P (1997) *Stuart and Sundeen's Mental Health Nursing: Principles and Practice*. Mosby-Wolfe. This is the British version of a classic American textbook. As its title suggests the book focuses on the principles and practice of mental health nursing care including chapters on concepts of mental health, models and theories, the therapeutic nurse–patient relationship, and service user perspectives. It also addresses the psychological, sociocultural, biological and legal and ethical context of mental health nursing, quality standards and supervision in professional practice. Chapters on health promotion, crisis theory and intervention, in-patient mental health care, liaison and consultation, and care for long-term clients are covered in the section on the principles of organizing care. The longest section of the book is all about applying the principles of mental health to nursing practice and includes many of the challenges that people with mental health problems are likely to experience with case studies and clear pointers on how mental health nurses can provide them with a high standard of care. Chapters include understanding suicidal behaviour, interventions with acutely ill patients, management of violence, drug and alcohol nursing, eating disorders, sexual health, child and adolescent and family mental health, care of older people, care of survivors of trauma, and forensic psychiatric nursing. Chapters on therapeutic approaches cover psychopharmacology, complementary therapies, behavioural psychotherapy, group work, schizophrenia family work. All the contributors are mental health nurses and experts in their field of practice. They provide a comprehensive textbook that will complement many training programmes and be a useful resource for students.

USEFUL WEBSITES

Centre for Evidence Based Mental Health – http://www.cebmh.com
Promoting and supporting the teaching and practice of evidence-based mental health care.

Chief Nursing Officer, Department of Health – www. dh.gov. uk/AboutUs/HeadsOfProfession/ChiefNursingOfficer/
Links to current information of interest to nurses.

KnowledgeShare – http://www.knowledgeshare.nhs.uk/index.htm
NHS information for evidence-based practice.

National Institute for Mental Health in England – http://www.nimhe.org.uk
NIMHE is responsible for supporting the implementation of positive change in mental health and mental health services.

Sainsbury Centre for Mental Health – http://www.scmh. org.uk
The Sainsbury Centre for Mental Health (SCMH) is a charity that works to improve the quality of life for people with severe mental health problems. It carries out research, development and training work to influence policy and practice in health and social care.

7

Perspectives on Learning Disability Nursing

Maureen Turner

INTRODUCTION

This chapter is intended as an introduction to learning disability nursing as a viable and credible career within the nursing profession. Learning disability nursing did not become part of the nursing profession until 1959 and is the least known of the four branches of nursing. This chapter will provide insight into how this branch of nursing has developed within the profession and how philosophies of care for people with learning disabilities have evolved and developed due to medical, social and political influences that have driven nurse education and practice. This chapter will provide insight into the contemporary knowledge, competencies and skills required by the learning disability nurse as stated by the Nursing and Midwifery Council (NMC) to meet the complex needs of people with learning disabilities. Thus the following areas will be considered:

- The medical, social and political influences that have governed care practice
- The development of learning disability nursing as a profession
- Public attitudes towards people with learning disability and their influence on care practice
- Changing care provision and nurse education
- Contemporary care practice and provision
- Skills attitudes and competencies required by the learning disability nurse
- The terminology used to describe people with learning disabilities

BACKGROUND TO THE DEVELOPMENT OF CONTEMPORARY CARE PRACTICES

To understand current practice, it is important to gain insight into the development of learning disability nursing as this will enable the reader to understand the changes that have led to contemporary practice within this branch of nursing. Throughout history, politicians, professionals from the fields of medicine, psychology, nursing and social work, as well as the general public through various pressure groups have debated the ways in which people with learning disabilities should be cared for. These opinions have influenced both service provision and care delivery.

Historically, people with learning disabilities were viewed negatively and often with suspicion by other members of society. Thus it is not surprising that people with a learning disability have acquired a negative image as words now considered derogatory in the English language have been used legislatively to describe people with learning disabilities. The Mental Deficiency Act (1913) used the terms 'idiot' and 'imbecile' to describe and define those who had a learning disability to distinguish them from those who had a mental health problem. Other terminology that would be considered equally derogatory, such as 'moral defective', has also been used legislatively and academically to describe the nature of a person's learning disability.

The Mental Health Act (1959) saw a change in the legislative language used to define the various classifications of learning disability and replaced words such as 'idiot' with 'subnormal', 'severely subnormal' or 'educationally subnormal'. At the time this was an attempt to remove the previously used derogatory labels, although the 1959 Act was not just about people with learning disabilities or changing labels. As attitudes changed the terminology in this act proved over time to be unhelpful and equally devaluing. In addition, learning disability nursing did not become part of the nursing profession until 1959 and was a direct result of the Act. Before this people with learning disabilities had been cared for in institutions by mainly unqualified staff who had no professional accountability, which implies devaluing care. These establishments eventually became hospitals managed by the National Health Service (NHS) with care being delivered by doctors and nurses.

Terminology also continued to change and eventually hospitals for the 'mentally subnormal' became known as hospitals for the 'mentally handicapped'. However, the aim of hospital care was to provide residential care and treatment; the care received in these overcrowded hospitals included *en bloc* treatment which was the only way that the basic needs could be met. Hospital staff could not realistically provide standards of care that upheld the privacy, dignity and individuality of the client, all of which are underpinning philosophies of contemporary practice.

The labelling of people with learning disabilities has changed consistently since the Mental Deficiency Act (1913) and Mental Health Act (1959) to meet the changing care philosophies, service provision, public perceptions of people with learning disabilities and more importantly, in acknowledgement of the voice of people with learning disabilities. It was their voice that made the decision to be collectively known as people (first) with learning disabilities (second).

By 1972, public, government and professionals attitudes were beginning to change towards the care of people with learning disabilities and this was followed by scrutiny of care practice by the Department of Health (DoH) which resulted in the publication of *Better Services for the Mentally*

Handicapped (1971) and the Jay Report (1979), both of which advocated care in the community for people with learning disabilities. These reports influenced and underpinned contemporary service provision, supporting people with learning disabilities to live in ordinary housing and live as normal a life as possible.

The change in service provision also changed the role of the learning disability nurse from one of providing little more than custodial care to enabling people with learning disabilities to live as independent a life as possible. This should be in an environment that maintains the privacy and dignity of each individual and provides support that enables each person to reach their maximum potential in all areas of their life. This change in care philosophy and practice was not only influenced by government reports and recommendations but also by the field of psychology. The publication of Wolfensberger's theories on normalization (1982) and social role valorization (1994), which also supported community living, had enormous impact on contemporary attitudes and practice. In addition, these theories described care philosophies that should underpin care delivery that promotes valuing people with learning disabilities and facilitates their value as individuals within society and the community in which they live. Contemporary practice is still based on the ideologies and philosophies of normalization and social role valorization.

The advent of registration for learning disability nurses held nurses accountable for their practice, and this had some influence on standards of care in the old hospitals for the 'mentally handicapped', but greater change was needed and this has evolved with the implementation of care in the community. Throughout history, practice has been influenced not only by government policy and society's views and the professions of medicine and psychology but also by the other branches of nursing.

Nursing models, which are theoretical frameworks on which to base care delivery, have been adapted and altered to meet the needs of this client group. Contemporary practice has led to learning disability nurses to develop special models and frameworks of care to meet the complex needs of people with learning disabilities.

Summary

- Many people with learning disabilities now living in the community lived in institutions and received little more than custodial care.
- Historically people with learning disabilities were viewed with suspicion and government acts such as the Mental Deficiency Act (1913) and the Mental Health Act (1959) assisted in segregating people with learning disabilities from society.
- People with learning disabilities were often feared.
- The care that they received was devaluing and degrading.

Reflective activity

Think of yourself as a person with a learning disability living in a hospital in an overcrowded ward. Write down all of the things that you take for granted that would not be available to you in one of these institutions.

Now write down how you might feel.

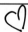

THE DEVELOPMENT OF THE QUALIFIED PRACTITIONER

The current term applied to a person with a learning disability receiving professional support is **client** and no longer patient, as the word patient implies a person who is sick. People with learning disabilities are not considered to be sick. Hence, the term client will be used throughout this chapter when describing contemporary practice. The recognition of the need for knowledgeable and skilled staff to deliver appropriate care to this client group equally has undergone many changes and has been influenced by the changing views of both government and society.

Attracting students into this branch of nursing has always been difficult and incentives in terms of pension have been used to encourage interest. There are several reasons why recruitment may have been difficult over the years. It is perhaps the least publicly known of the four branches of nursing and historically those with learning disabilities and their carers have had a negative image among the general public. This has perhaps been due to a lack of information generally being made available about the needs of people who have a learning disability and the role of the learning disability nurse in caring for this client group. Part of the role of the learning disability nurse is to encourage a positive image of people with a learning disability to promote their successful integration into normal community life.

The influence resulting from the use of labels has not only come from government legislation but also from the field of psychology and pressure groups in society. After the introduction of the Mental Health Act (1959) attitudes were already changing towards people with learning disabilities and their care. The idea that people with learning disabilities could benefit from an ordinary life has been gaining momentum since the days of the *Better Services for the Mentally Handicapped* Report (1971), The National Development Group Report (1978), the Jay Report (1979) and Wolfensberger's publications on normalization theory (1982) and media coverage by pressure groups in society.

INFLUENCES DRIVING THE LEARNING DISABILITY NURSING CURRICULUM

The influences discussed above led to the change in the pre-registration nursing syllabus in 1982, which ceased to use the term subnormal and severely subnormal and instead encompassed the notion of this client group as people first and handicapped second. Consequently a qualifying nurse registered as an RNMH (Registered Nurse for the Mentally Handicapped) and not RNMS. Currently, a qualifying nurse registers as an RNLD.

The Mental Health Act 1983 equally changed the terminology in keeping with the changing views of society, the fields of psychology, nursing and medicine. This point demonstrates that care philosophy and provision have not been static and that the influence for change has not been purely

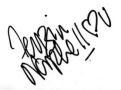

government-directed but has changed with the views of other professions and society.

Although professional registration for learning disability nurses was not introduced until 1959 a syllabus for caring for 'mental defectives' was developed in 1923. This saw the beginning of the separation between those with mental ill health and those with learning disabilities. However, the separation of these two patient groups was formalized with the introduction of the National Assistance Act 1948 and the development of the NHS. Specialist hospitals cared for people with a wide range of learning disabilities and, as stated above, were often buildings that had previously been workhouses.

Summary

There has been radical change in care delivery for people with learning disabilities and learning disability practice has changed from providing custodial care to:

- enabling people with learning disabilities to live in the community
- promoting the independence of people with learning disabilities
- teaching people with learning disabilities the skills of ordinary living
- promoting a positive image of people with learning disabilities.

Reflective activity

Write down the skills that you think a person with a learning disability will need to be taught to live as independently as possible in the community. Use your previous list to consider all of the things that you take for granted. This will enable you to think of how learning disability nurses plan care interventions.

CHANGES IN NURSE EDUCATION

The Briggs report on nurse education (1972) first questioned the need for carers of people with learning disabilities to be nurses as these people are not sick. This report recommended that this branch of nursing should no longer be part of the nursing profession and that another kind of carer could provide the care required by people with learning disabilities. The report was produced at the same time as the government commissioned a report known as *Better Services for the Mentally Handicapped*, which was published in 1971.

The main recommendations of the 1971 report were to prevent people with a learning disability being cared for in hospital but for adequate and appropriate support services to be provided in the community to enable the person with a learning disability to be cared for in their own home. It also recommended that local authority take lead responsibility for assessing appropriate care and providing adequate services.

In 1978 the Department of Health commissioned the National Development Group to investigate the standards of care in hospitals. This report also advocated people with learning disabilities being cared for in much smaller groups and where possible in normal housing. It also recommended that children with a learning disability should not be cared for in long-stay institutions. The Jay Report (1979) quickly followed and also recommended that people with a learning disability should be cared for in the community, but added that people with learning disabilities did not require registered nurses to care for them.

Each of these reports influenced the closure of the large hospitals for people with learning disabilities and provision of more appropriate care in the community. These reports collectively have driven learning disability nursing to cross the boundaries of health and social care, and, in part, influenced the 1982 syllabus, which had greater focus on meeting the social care needs of people with learning disabilities. Hence another change in terminology: people with learning disabilities became increasingly referred to as clients rather than patients. The curriculum for learning disability nurses changed from a medical model of care to a model of social care that focused on promoting independence by teaching clients self-help skills and social skills. This included accessing community facilities, interacting with others in the community and acquiring the skills of daily living that ordinary people take for granted.

The continued evolvement of the curriculum into Project 2000 (United Kingdom Central Council for Nursing, Midwifery and Health Visiting (UKCC)) has more clearly identified the role of the learning disability nurse within current health care facilitation.

Moves towards improvement

Although hospital care for many years had focused on meeting the basic physical needs of patients, attempts had been made to teach people with learning disabilities self-help skills in addition to changes in behaviour that would be considered challenging. The introduction of behavioural intervention techniques, which is reinforcing behaviour that is desirable (based on Skinner's theories of operant conditioning (cited in Glassman, 2003), meant that nurses could make a difference to the lives of people with a learning disability.

Behavioural psychology had been the major influence on clinical practice at this time and knowledge of behavioural psychology, although modified, continues to have an influence in both skill teaching and in attempting to change the challenging behaviour of people with learning disabilities. Promoting their independence through the development of self-help and social skills, as well as changing behaviour that may be considered challenging, can change the destiny for many people with learning disabilities and give them hope of returning to normal community living.

As with any profession, change is not immediate and as it evolves the implications of change and the need for frameworks and guidelines become apparent. Although at this time behavioural intervention therapy was viewed by the profession as a radical move towards promoting the independence and individuality of the client it appears that nurses and other professionals were doing things *to* the client rather than *with* the client.

The role of the learning disability nurse in contemporary practice is much more about working with the client and their carers in partnership, to provide choice and empower the person with a learning disability to have control over their own lives and destiny while working within the NMC's code of conduct (see Appendix 2).

Summary

Learning disability nursing skill base has changed to:

- teaching people with learning disabilities self-help skills based on behavioural theory
- teaching people with learning disabilities social skills
- enabling people with learning disabilities to access normal community facilities
- enabling people with learning disabilities to live as independently as possible.

Reflective activity

Write down one self-help skill like washing or dressing yourself and break this down into small steps to be able to teach a person with a learning disability that skill. Look at the NMC's competencies and match these skills to those outcomes.

Contemporary practice

This evolving role of the learning disability nurse has been influenced by changing ideology that questioned not only the practice of learning disability nurse but also the very nature of service provision. It created radical change in both the living environments of people with learning disabilities and the philosophy of care underpinning the practice delivered by the registered nurse. The normalization theory states that people with learning disabilities should:

- lead as a normal life as possible
- live in ordinary housing
- have access to social and leisure facilities enjoyed by the general public
- have access to normal health care facilities enjoyed by the general public
- gain access to employment
- develop meaningful relationships.

In conclusion, having greater choice and control over their lives.

This change in care philosophy created the need for clinical leaders, service providers and registered learning disability nurses to reflect on their practice and return control of people's lives to the individual by working in partnership with clients and their families. The change in care philosophy was introduced gradually: as with any system of radical change one regimen does not automatically replace another. Consequently the influence of behavioural therapy continues to coexist alongside contemporary care ideologies in varying degrees of modification, particularly in relation to teaching skills and promoting independence.

The notion of positive reinforcement is still evident in contemporary practice although this is encompassed into care plans far more as a shared decision with clients than as the notion of manipulating clients by the use of reinforcement. However, it must be noted that enabling people with learning disabilities to be more independent is viewed by the profession as a prerequisite to community living. The coexistence of these two principles of care, although on the surface two extremes, was implemented to achieve the one desired goal of community living. This radical change in thought and attitudes towards the care of people with learning disabilities has been continuously driven by the notion that people with learning disabilities could benefit from living as ordinary a life as possible with the same expectations as all others in society.

Consequently, normalization and social role valorization have become the foundation of the learning disability pre-registration nursing curriculum. Practitioners are able to demonstrate through appropriate care delivery that people with a learning disability are people first and disabled second. Both service providers and registered nurses have a responsibility to develop individualized plans and packages of care to meet the total needs of the client by providing a seamless service.

WORKING WITH OTHER PROFESSIONALS

Caring for people with learning disabilities living in the community requires a registered nurse to acquire skills to work autonomously as a safe and competent practitioner and also as an effective practitioner working as part of a multi-professional team. Learning disability nurses are held accountable for their professional conduct and competency by the NMC. Due to the multi-professional nature of care delivery it is difficult to measure quantitatively the contribution the learning disability nurse makes to client care. However, the learning disability nurse has a key role in ensuring that the contribution of each professional meets the total needs of the client.

The *Continuing the Commitment Report* (DoH, 1995) supported multi-professional working and recognized the need for learning disability nurses to work in partnership with other professionals, agencies and carers. This is particularly important since the introduction of normalization, social role valorization and the move to community living as the care of people with learning disabilities has become the responsibility of a diversity of agencies. It has meant that the registered learning disability nurse is required to maintain the unique skills of caring directly for the client while working in partnership with the person, family, other professionals and care workers to provide care that meets the total needs of the individual.

Multi-professional care is a necessity if clients are to receive the level of support that is required for them to gain maximum independence and quality of life from community living. This means working with social services, educators of people with special needs, doctors, physiotherapists, occupational therapists, speech and language therapists, psychologists and the independent sector providing residential care. These working partnerships facilitate the provision of a seamless service intended to meet the total and complex needs of people with learning disabilities. The learning disability nurse has a key role to play in both co-ordinating and delivering care.

In order to fulfil the nurse's role in a new and evolving service the new pre-registration nursing curriculum incorporates biology, psychology, sociology, information technology and nursing practice to equip newly qualified staff to appropriately meet the complex health and social care needs of the person with learning disabilities. The knowledge and skills of the learning disability nurse include (see Appendix 1):

- communication with people who are not able to communicate verbally
- empowering people with learning disabilities to be self-advocating
- enabling people with learning disabilities to develop meaningful relationships
- promoting the health and well-being of people with complex health and social care needs
- managing and changing difficult behaviour
- promoting independence to the maximum potential of the individual
- ensuring that the education and training needs of the individual are met
- assessing need and planning care to promote quality of life for the individual
- ensuring that care delivery meets both the health and social care needs of the individual client.

According to Cullen (cited in *Continuing the Commitment Report*, DoH, 1995) application of concepts such as normalization, social role valorization, community care and empowerment have become so much part of best practice for learning disability nurses as well as other professionals that they may be considered dominant ideologies.

Learning disability nursing is not only about underpinning practice with the recognized ideologies and philosophies, it is also about the attainment of skills. To practice effectively, a wide range of clinical, behavioural and attitudinal skills are required. Having the knowledge and skill to teach and develop the communication skills of the individual to enable them to make their needs known can make a huge difference to their lives, promoting their self-esteem and self-worth.

Thus communication and interpersonal skills are a major focus of the learning disability curriculum and nurses who have difficulties with both communication and interpersonal skills are not going to interact effectively with clients who have a learning disability, their family or other carers.

Summary

Learning disability nurses need to be able to:

- empower people with learning disabilities to advocate for themselves and make choices
- work across the boundaries of health care and social care
- develop communication skills to work effectively with the clients, their carers and their families
- use a range of therapeutic interventions that promote the independence, health and well-being of the individual with learning disabilities
- facilitate the opportunity for people with learning disabilities to develop social networks
- provide the opportunity for people with learning disabilities to develop and maintain meaningful relationships.

These competencies are required by the NMC (Appendix 1).

Reflective activity

Write down the skills you feel that you already have to achieve the above and then list the ones that you feel you need to develop.

MAINTAINING MAXIMUM HEALTH AND WELL-BEING

The learning disability nurse working in today's service has a key role in the total health facilitation of the individual with learning disabilities, by promoting the maximum health and well-being of that individual. Maximum health and well-being is not just concerned with the physical health of the individual but also the mental well-being of the person.

Mental health

According to Raghavan *et al.* (2004) prevalence of mental ill health is higher among people with learning disabilities than in the normal population and have an increased likelihood of having depression because their lifestyle is much more likely to result in lowered self-esteem and self-worth.

The skill and knowledge of the learning disability nurse enables them not only to recognize mental ill health and intervene appropriately but also to prevent mental health problems. This is achieved in part by increasing the autonomy and control an individual has over their own life as these increase the individual's own self-value and self-worth. The greater one's independence the less likely a person is to become depressed. It is equally important that nurses understand the theories of institutionalization and the effects that depersonalization may have had in contributing to the wide range of mental disorders in people with learning disabilities.

People with a learning disability have the right to access the same treatment as the wider general population. It is not solely recognition of the illness and care that is the duty of the registered learning disability nurse, but it is also necessary for the responsible nurse to evaluate the effectiveness of any treatment given and provide support for the client during the illness. For registered nurses to be confident and competent to be able to do this student nurses need to acquire an academic understanding of the theories of psychology and mental ill health. This theoretical understanding is reinforced through experience in a range of practice settings that care for those people with learning disabilities who also have mental health problems.

The aim of specialist care for those people with learning disabilities who also have mental health problems is to provide treatment and rehabilitation so that they may return to an ordinary life in the community. This may mean that the community learning disability nurse continues to support the client after discharge to prevent further re-admissions.

Challenging behaviour

Some people with learning disabilities exhibit high levels of challenging behaviour and it is the role of the learning disability nurse to understand and manage that behaviour. According to Repp *et al.* (1989) challenging behaviour is most effectively managed when treatment is based on the hypothesis of its cause. The learning disability nurse working in contemporary practice in this much specialized area is required to have a sound knowledge of the biological, psychological and sociological theories that underpin the motivation for challenging behaviour to understand, manage and treat challenging behaviour effectively.

Excellent communication skills are of paramount importance when interacting with clients who challenge their carers and the service. The care philosophy underpinning practice when working with this group of people is still to value the individual and promote a positive image of this client group in the community in which they live. The skill base of the registered learning disability nurse is complex as in addition to recognizing and managing an individual's mental health problems and challenging behaviour they are also required to have the knowledge and skill to meet the complex physical needs of the person with a learning disability.

Physical health care needs

According to Tait and Genders (2002) people with learning disabilities have more complex physical needs than the normal population. Those people with profound learning and physical disabilities may require the intervention of specialist clinical skills. For example, due to their profound physical disability a few clients have eating difficulties that require mechanical aids such as percutaneous endoscopic gastrostomy (PEG) feeding. It is necessary that staff undertaking such procedures are competent and confident to always maintain the safety and well-being of the client. This requires greater skill than just being able to go through the motions of being able to perform the task. There is equally a need for the practitioner, who is accountable, to acquire a wider knowledge of the implications of such procedures and to be able to act in accordance with the policies and frameworks that govern practice to always ensure the client's safety and well-being.

Clients who do have complex health and social care needs are extremely vulnerable and are often totally dependent on their carers to recognize when their physical or mental state of health has changed. The ability to observe and interpret each individual's state of wellness requires a specialist skill, especially as many clients with multiple needs are often unable to articulate their desires, needs and feelings verbally. Caring for this client group is developed through a continuum of knowledge and skills that encompass both the tasks and the art of nursing.

Summary

To manage, treat and meet the mental health needs, challenging behaviour and physical health needs of people with learning disabilities the learning disability nurse requires a knowledge of:

- theories of biology, psychology, sociology and the aetiology of learning disability
- effective and appropriate care interventions
- clinical nursing skills
- the roles of other professionals in meeting the complex health care needs of people with learning disabilities.

Reflective activity

The learning disability nurse requires knowledge as well as skills. Write down the topics that you think you will be required to study at diploma level to underpin practice with sound evidence.

ASSESSING, PLANNING AND IMPLEMENTING CARE

Individual needs are not identified on the basis of assumption but on accurate assessment. This is not merely a check list of problems, it is information about all internal and external influences that may have affected an individual's life.

The learning disability nurse working in today's service has a key role in the total health facilitation of the individual with learning disabilities. It is the specific role of the learning disability nurse

to collect accurate information and analyse the data collected during the assessment that will use this information to plan effective care. It is through accurate observation and interpretation of the information collected that the knowledge and skill of the learning disability nurse facilitates the development of appropriate care plans to meet the complex health and social care needs of the client and improve quality of life for the individual.

Nurses carrying out assessments and developing care plans have to remember that all information concerning the client is relevant. In addition to collecting information relating to the physical and mental health state of the client other factors such as age, gender, previous life experiences and the cause of the person's learning disability are important. For example, Cosgrave *et al.* (1999) clearly inform us that there is an association between Down's syndrome and Alzheimer's disease; therefore it is important that consideration is given to this fact if an elderly client with Down's syndrome presents with an altered health state. Equally it is important that all care interventions are age appropriate as it is demeaning and devaluing to treat an adult as a child. This is not an exhaustive list and the skill of the learning disability nurse is to be able consider each area of a person's life that will impact on their current health status.

The ability to synthesize the information collected during the assessment process and make accurate judgement relies on the knowledge of the nurse carrying out the assessment. The pre-registration nursing curriculum includes a range of academic subjects that provide students with the appropriate knowledge which will enable them to consider the relationship between a person's environment, lifestyle, skills, and physical and mental well-being. This same knowledge ultimately provides the competent practitioner with the information required to develop appropriate care plans to overcome any barriers to maximum health and well-being.

Planning care

This approach to care planning – considering all aspects of a person's life rather than a list of problems – prevents care from being delivered in a compartmentalized fashion which may mean that some of the client's individual needs may be omitted. Equally, nurses need to have a self-awareness of their own limitations in terms of both skills and knowledge to guarantee that clients benefit from the diversity of knowledge possessed by the care team during the care planning process.

In addition to gaining knowledge and skills in communication, care planning and the promotion of advocacy it is essential that the curriculum addresses the ethical issues involved in caring for such a vulnerable group of people. The learning disability pre-registration curriculum includes a variety of challenging topics that enable the practitioner to consider the ethical implications of their practice. Consequently, any care intervention designed to change any area of a client's life that may be considered intrusive has to be carefully analysed in terms of the ethical implications.

Practitioners should be able to justify how the change may improve the client's quality of life and enable the person to become more independent. Any form of treatment or care intervention designed to promote independence invariably necessitates some form of intimate interaction with the person; therefore consideration has to be given to the client's wishes and desires. However, gaining consent for such interaction can be difficult when caring for people who may have little or no verbal communication. The responsibility for ensuring that the client is consenting relies on the skill of the registered practitioner and their knowledge of the client to interpret that consent has been given.

Summary

The competencies required by the learning disability nurse are to be able to:

- assess, plan and implement care to meet the total needs of clients
- work in partnership with clients and their carers to develop care plans that encompass the client's choices
- consider the ethical implications of care interventions.

The learning disability nurse is constantly faced with a wide range of ethical dilemmas that require the expertise to make decisions in relation to care practice that are genuinely in the client's best interest.

Reflective activity

Consider a variety of ways that you could involve a person with learning disabilities in their care without using verbal communication. Also consider what you think some of the ethical issues surrounding learning disability practice might be.

PHILOSOPHIES OF CARE

Care philosophies informing practice have for some considerable time emphasized the need for people with learning disabilities to receive individualized care. The competent practitioner will always have to reflect on their interactions with clients and their families to be sure that they have taken into account the ethical, cultural and spiritual needs of the client and their family, even if this means the most favourable care intervention cannot be implemented without causing offence. Practitioners cannot claim competence and expertise from the length of time spent in clinical practice but need to be able to justify their practice from a sound evidence base. This means that registered nurses have an obligation to remain up to date in terms of contemporary research and published evidence.

Pre-registration student nurses are taught throughout the programme to critique and analyse research and judge the value of specific research studies as being valid and credible to underpin clinical practice. Care intervention based on sound evidence and research provides registered nurses with an academic justification for care delivery that is open to question and scrutiny. It is equally important for learning disability nurses to be able to undertake research to ensure that contemporary practice continues to develop and evolve. Consequently all pre-registration nursing programmes include the research process and methodology within the curriculum.

Evidence-based practice

There is a need to research and analyse clinical practice and care delivery carried out by learning disability nurses to augment the credibility and viability of learning disability practitioners. It is through the articulation of research developed from within the profession that the unique contribution that learning disability nurses make to the care of their clients becomes evident. It has been of benefit to people with learning disabilities and the profession to have been so closely scrutinized and questioned prior to the advent of community care. There is equally a need for care delivery to be less influenced by other professionals than it has been historically and for learning disability nurses to publicize evidence and more clearly demonstrate the diversity of their role in meeting the total needs of the clients.

Summary

The learning disability nurse needs to plan care:

- based on sound evidence from a wide range of literature
- based on contemporary philosophies.

Reflective activity

Because learning disability nursing practice has been influenced by other professions and clinical practice is centred around multi-professional working, consider the various sources of literature that you could access to help you to develop a sound knowledge base.

It is evident from this chapter that the care of people with learning disabilities and the profession of learning disability nursing have undergone radical change over the past 30 years. The scrutiny into clinical practice has constantly provided the medium for individual clinicians to reflect on their own practice as well as for managers and nurse educators to consider care from the point of view of the organization, which has to be a positive step rather than a negative one.

LEARNING DISABILITY NURSING IN THE FUTURE

The latest government report *Valuing People* (DoH, 2001) undoubtedly acknowledges that the rights of people with learning disabilities are the same as for any other member of society and include the right to employment, housing, education and general health care. The report equally acknowledges that people with learning disabilities have perhaps not enjoyed the same standards of general health care as the normal population. The future role of the learning disability nurse may well be in facilitating access to general health care services with a view to this client group gaining quality of life through maximum health and well-being. This will require student nurses following all four nursing pathways to gain insight into the lives of people with learning disabilities so that they may care for them appropriately in general health care settings.

Student nurses following the learning disability branch programme will need to be provided with the knowledge and skills that prepare them to work in flexible and changing health and social care arenas to meet the individual needs of people with learning disabilities. It is through rigorous academic and practice assessments, which measure if the learning outcomes of the programme have been met, that students will develop the personal and professional competence they need to demonstrate their fitness for practice.

The curriculum's learning outcomes will also need to be constantly evaluated to ensure that new government proposals and contemporary issues are incorporated to prepare student nurses to be competent practitioners in tomorrow's wide-ranging care settings and support services. The future for learning disability nurses appears to be focused on meeting the health care needs of people with learning disabilities and ensuring that all of their health care needs are met. This will require learning disability nurses to be far more community based and they will need to continue to work with a wide range of professionals. Nurses will also be required to undertake programmes in higher education at post-registration level to continue to lead the profession in meeting the changing service demands.

CONCLUSION

The skills and competencies of the registered learning disability nurse cannot always be articulated in terms of tasks but are expressed in a wide range of complex skills that are both behavioural and attitudinal. The future of the learning disability nurse continues to be to work across professional boundaries facilitating maximum health and well-being of people with learning disabilities, supporting this client group to be their own advocates and live a quality of life that is expected by others in society.

GLOSSARY

In the context of this chapter the meanings of the following words are described:

Advocate	Person who acts on their own behalf, or if a person with a learning disability has an advocate, this person would intercede on their behalf
Behavioural psychology	Understanding and changing behaviour by observing environmental reinforcements
Down's syndrome	Chromosomal abnormality resulting in varying degrees of learning disability. The risk of this disorder increases with maternal age
Eugenics	Study of improving the human race
Normalization	Means being treated in a way that an individual is happy to accept and is not about being 'made normal' (Chisholm, cited in Shanley E and Starrs T (eds) (1993) *Learning Disability: a handbook of care.* Edinburgh, Churchill Livingstone p. 41)
Social role valorization	Universal principle on which services for those with learning disabilities are based

REFERENCES

Briggs Report (1972) *Report of the Committee on Nursing.* London: HMSO.

Cosgrave MP, Tyrell J, Carron M, Gill BA, Lawlar (1999) Age at onset of dementia and age of menopause in women with Down's syndrome. *Journal of Intellectual Disability Research* 43:446–65.

Department of Health and Social Security (1971) *Better Services for the Mentally Handicapped.* London: HMSO.

Department of Health (1995) *Continuing the Commitment Report.* London: HMSO.

Department of Health (2001) *Valuing People. A new strategy for learning disability for the 21st century.* London: HMSO.

Glassman W (2003) *Approaches to Psychology*, 3rd edn. Buckinghamshire: Open University Press, p. 120.

Jay Report (1979) *Report of the committee of enquiry into mental handicap and nursing care.* London: HMSO.

Mental Deficiency Act (1913) Cited in: Morris P (1969) *Put Away. A social study for the mentally retarded.* London: Routledge and Kegan Paul, pp. 22–3.

Mental Health Act 1959. London: HMSO.

Mental Health Act 1983. London: HMSO.

National Assistance Act (1948) Cited in: Morris P (1969) *Put Away. A social study for the mentally retarded.* London: Routledge and Kegan Paul, p. 257.

National Development Group report (1978) London: HMSO.

Raghavan R, Marshall M, Lockwood A, Duggan L (2004) Assessing the needs of people with learning disability and mental illness: development of the learning disability version of the Cardinal Needs Schedule. *Journal of Intellectual Disability Research* 48:25–36.

Registered Nurse for the Mentally Handicapped syllabus (1982) UKCC.

Repp A, Felce C, Barton E, Lyle D (1989) Basing the treatment of stereotypic and self injurious behaviour on the hypotheses of their cause. *Journal of Applied Behavioural Analysis* 21:281–9.

Tait T, Genders N (2002) *Caring for People with Learning Disabilities.* London: Arnold pp. 55–60.

United Kingdom Central Council for Nursing, Midwifery and Health Visiting. *Project 2000 A new preparation for practice.* London: UKCC.

Wolfensberger W (1982) Social role valorisation. A proposed term for the principle of normalisation. *Mental Retardation* 21:234–9.

Wolfensberger W (1994) An analysis of the client role from a social role valorisation perspective. *The International Social Role Valorization Journal* 1(1):3–8.

ANNOTATED FURTHER READING

Tait T, Genders N (2002) *Caring for People with Learning Disabilities.* London: Arnold. This is an extremely useful book for students on the foundations of learning disability practice.

Gates B (1997) *Learning Disabilities,* 3rd edn. Edinburgh: Churchill Livingstone. This book covers many issues related to contemporary practice.

Jukes M, Bollard M (2003) *Contemporary Learning Disability.* Dinton Quay: Health Care Limited. This book includes a wide range of issues surrounding contemporary practice for nurses working in learning disabilities including inter-professional working, valuing people and the complex health needs of people with learning disabilities.

Recommended journals

Journal of Learning Disabilities for Nursing Health and Social Care
Nursing Times
Learning Disability Practice.

USEFUL WEBSITES

British Institute of Learning Disabilities. www.bild.org.uk
www.Dh.gov.uk/PolicyAndGuidance/HealthandSocialcare Topics/Learning Disabilities/fs/en
Learning Disability Practice. www.learningdisabilitypractice.co.uk

8

Support Systems for Student Nurses

Nick Salter

INTRODUCTION

This chapter aims to enlighten you about the personal challenges that you may face during a course of study. Support can offer the chance to cope better with those challenges. The nature of support will be explained and the importance of support systems and the possible benefits will be discussed. It is hoped that when armed with this information, you will feel more able to solve problems and will look forward to the changes and challenges that lie ahead.

Many people give support in different situations and it takes place in both formal and informal styles. Various types of support are needed at different times but sometimes support does not happen. This may be due to a feeling of weakness or failure or simply not knowing what help is on offer and from whom it can be sought. There is a range of support systems that are an essential part of student experience. Then there is additional support available if other problems occur, for example, homesickness, debt or problems with accommodation. As a result of reading this chapter it is hoped that you will understand what can be achieved and to whom you might turn for help. At the end of this chapter you will find a list of useful websites. These will help you to answer these questions.

When contemplating a university-based course of study there are so many choices and decisions to make:

- Which course?
- Which university do I choose?
- Do I want to leave home and live independently?
- What kind of accommodation will I look for?
- Can I afford to live independently?
- Will I have to gain paid employment to supplement my bursary?
- Will I have to buy lots of expensive books?

There are many more questions to ask and decisions to make and you might be able to answer them more easily with some help.

Reflective activity

This first activity aims to start you thinking about yourself. As caring people, we so often put others' needs first and forget ourselves. Under the following headings, make a list of your ideas about these new situations you will have to get used to when you start your course:

Getting to know your way around
Adjusting to working in practice placements
Fitting into new groups or teams
Managing your study time
Managing your finances

Perceptions of student support

Your perceptions of the benefits of support at university may have developed from your own experiences at school or from experiences that your peers have shared with you, either recently or in the distant past. Positive experiences with, for example school teachers, could induce a belief that future relationships with lecturers will be beneficial. However, previous negative experiences could work against a possible successful student–lecturer relationship. When at school we often saw the teachers if things went wrong. A summons to 'the office' created doubt and fear. We might have thought 'Why me?' or 'What does he want me for?' Lecturers though, like teachers, are well able to dispense praise; they like nothing more. They enjoy helping students solve problems, guiding them and rewarding good work.

Actually, as a lecturer, it is very easy to become enthusiastic about the outcome of support. The whole object of support is to help students. Support should ease your development and passage through the educational experience. A lecturer might help simply by listening to what you have to say. Advice could take the form of a direction, or a course of action that you could take. You may need persuasion or help towards making a decision. A lecturer might support a decision or your behaviour as being acceptable, praise you for your achievements and reassure you to help maintain your effort.

Outcomes of support

Students can achieve a level of **re-assurance** (as an outcome) (Teasdale, 1989) by simply knowing that support is available; that there is someone or something to turn to. Feelings of success are very positive motivators and these can come from feedback from assignments, placement reports, tutorials and exam successes. Motivation is a great driving force. Sometimes students need encouragement to seek feedback and advice from lecturers and this can also come from peers. Often students learn together from shared experiences and the feeling of partnership can strengthen the desire to do well for each other and learning that takes place together can seem more valuable.

Personal support can help maintain positive behaviour and therefore learning. It can encourage the development of both personal and professional skills. So often, support attempts to enthuse students into action or decision-making. At times, when a student becomes unhappy or depressed, clarity of vision is lost. Support will attempt to re-orientate the student to reality. This process can be a difficult one and students may need many sources of support. The student may be seeking some sort of consolation or comfort during times of trouble. Symptoms of suffering are often difficult to alleviate and are often easier to spot in someone else rather than oneself.

Supporters also help by enlivening the mind and creating a sense of cheer; feelings that create hope and purpose in the mind. These positive states can help, when for example, study behaviour may need adapting to meet new situations, a change in the level of assessment, a new placement for practical experiences or when reactions to events requires new preparations for the future. Plans and arrangements for future experiences may need careful consideration and timely, effective support may make some positive difference.

One outcome of support is the creation of independence. There would be nothing gained by supporters who wish to make students dependent upon their advice. It should be obvious then, that a significant amount of responsibility for self-determination depends on willpower. As the Nursing and Midwifery Council code of conduct (NMC, 2002; see Appendix 2) indicates in section 6 you will, as a registered nurse, be responsible for your own development, so during your course you will need to develop your ability to be responsible for your own actions. As a student, you will work under the supervision of registered nurses. However, your aim should be to practise safely and effectively without direct supervision and maintain your own knowledge and the skills required wherever you practice.

Summary

This discussion has described support in a general sense with the aim to enthuse you to view support in a positive manner. The following sections discuss some of the common reasons why students might seek support or to put it another way, some of the many needs students may experience during training. A further section discusses possible sources of support.

POSSIBLE CHALLENGES TO CONSIDER

Changes to accommodation

Leaving home can be an upheaval, leaving a familiar environment, routine, people with whom you live and friends. The need to learn how to perform domestic activities might be a major new experience that could seem daunting. On the other hand, changes might be preferable to present arrangements and new experiences may be those that have been looked forward to for some time. Many students, especially mature students, choose to stay at home. This can produce savings on expenses as well as reducing the need for change. As the need to study changes and the time that you will spend at home changes, some allowances need to be made by you and all who live with you. Often, students talk about the notion that their families and friends go through the course with them so even your family and friends could be making some sacrifices.

Arranging accommodation itself might be a new experience and advice is available from, e.g. university accommodation officers, housing agencies and students' unions. You will want to live in secure, safe and comfortable housing and some universities actually guarantee accommodation for your first year of study especially if you are from overseas. When you receive you final offer from your chosen university, you will receive a form P76. This is your Accommodation Preference Form and it must be returned within seven days if you are from the UK.

Living in university halls of residence is an experience some students relish whereas others prefer to avoid it. It is a matter of taste and no two halls are the same. Try to visit prospective halls and talk to resident students for their views, then make up your mind. The quality of accommodation worries a lot of students and their parents when, for example, there has been no prior viewing. There is a tendency to make friendship groups quickly and often, small groups move halls to be with each other. Some leave halls and rent accommodation together to give them a greater sense of independence. Private accommodation is usually available and the local advice centre, accommodation officer or the student union are all available to give advice. Many students enjoy living with other student nurses because they gain a lot of peer support regarding course issues even if they are living with students in another year group or branch speciality.

There are some very useful internet sites that offer sound advice. Try www.merlinhelpsstudents.com – this site offers advice about accommodation, advice on renting in the private sector, safety issues, contracts, types of tenancy, deposits, university lodgings and the benefits of staying at home. It may be worth approaching an accommodation agency. Look at local papers and their websites, notice boards and perhaps actually look at the student housing on offer. This is often an option on university open days. Another helpful internet site is www.connexions-direct.com – this site displays advice about housing, i.e. student accommodation, housing benefits, moving out/leaving home, and more.

Inventories of contents should always be checked upon entering the accommodation for the first time. This should include an inspection of any damage already present and although accommodation should be in an acceptable condition, what constitutes acceptable is open to debate. If you need to make a complaint try to be objective and fair and be prepared to compromise at least until you settle in. Over time, you will discover alternatives and avenues to getting changes made.

One of the fears for some students, especially those who have not lived away from home before, is homelessness. Occasionally accommodation is arranged too late for the agency or accommodation officer to give any advanced notice of location. It is something to keep a wary eye on. Check the location and type of accommodation on offer at the interview stage and make a note to enquire about its availability if information does not arrive when you expect it.

Mature students may need to adapt their lifestyle to meet their need to study effectively. This may mean simply that furniture is moved around or a desk brought into the house. This may affect how the house or a particular room is used. A dining room may become a temporary office. The family will experience the changes and may not enjoy the encroachment into their space. The way changes are made and rationalized may be more important than the physical alterations themselves.

Managing your finances

Most students find it difficult to spend money wisely. The lack of money might occur due to poor **budgeting**. You may not have had much experience of handling money for food, clothing, accommodation and study expenses, paying bills, fees and living on a limited budget. Bank managers, student services departments, student loan departments, parents and spouses are there to give help if necessary so do not think that you are on your own if you get into difficulties. Financial problems are best managed as soon as they become apparent rather than when debt has become uncontrolled.

The amount of money student nurses gain from their bursary is easily spent. Many students are in debt to banks or building societies. Many feel indebted to their parents or supporters and this can produce an intense feeling of guilt. However, more students these days accept that debt is just another consequence of being a university student. The issue here is that you may experience the need to seek employment to supplement your income (see section on working while you are a student). This might be to fund loan repayments or to help pay for basic requirements such as food and accommodation expenses or childcare fees. Christmas and holiday times produce special demands on finances especially for students who may be parents or carers, and mature students who may have family-related commitments that younger students do not experience. These might be related to partners' unemployment or business-related expenses.

New students may not fully appreciate the important issue of travelling expenses. While at school or college, the institution, parents and friends often arrange transport. It may have been subsidized by the institution or your parents. However, when at university, you may bear the cost of transport for the first time. The burden of responsibility may also be an unknown quantity. The expense, time and frustrations of car breakdowns, missing buses or trains may add to the mounting stresses. Try to make yourself aware of the chance for previous travel reimbursements or the presence of any university student hardship funds and how you can access them. Many internet sites offer advice on bursary issues, finance and counselling services; see the NMC website (www. nmc-uk.org). Have a look at websites for cheaper travel offers. Check also with your university if uniforms are provided. Some branches of nursing do not require uniforms, for example, learning disabilities and fewer uniforms may be issued during the common foundation programme.

Being in control of personal finances reduces the deleterious effects of financial hardship. This facilitates a greater focus on study and the positive effects of employment and personal management that can help improve a sense of self-esteem.

Managing your learning

The start of any course or even a module of study produces a plethora of new information to be understood and integrated into new routines. Most peers will be in a similar position so talk with them to see what sense they make of it all and to facilitate awareness that you are not alone in your feelings and thoughts.

Using your initiative for organizing your time might be a novel experience. You will need to accept that you are responsible for your learning. Lecturers have a responsibility to teach but they cannot learn for you. In practice, it means preparing for lectures, for example, gaining insights and motivation from the lecturers and reading around the subject thus gaining further information to help you form opinions and alter your thinking about what has been heard and seen.

There are some potential difficulties in relation to resources. Obtaining books and journal articles can take a long time and can cost money. There will probably be insufficient books in most libraries for all students to be able to borrow copies of the same book at the same time; so use the short loan and recall systems. Photocopying costs money and this is an expense that needs to be anticipated. Try to plan around the times when there will be heavy demand on certain key texts. You could request and save book tokens from birthdays, for example. Only buy a book that you have looked through and that seems essential, for example a dictionary, anatomy and physiology book, key psychology and sociology texts might be recommended. The use of the internet has expanded greatly and you may be experienced in its use. There may be IT skills sessions arranged for you if you wish to become more proficient. Gain some experience in the use of various search engines, databases and electronic journals; library support staff will be useful. Always remember to share information and resources with peers as this can save time and money, and it will nurture symbiotic relationships.

Meeting deadlines, handing in assignments and getting behind with work often causes stress. **Time management** can be a skill that takes years of practise. Setting goals by working back from assessment deadlines is essential. Remember that lecturers, peers and students who are more experienced can offer advice and encouragement so discuss any difficulties you have with them. If all else fails lecturers could agree to give extensions to assignment deadlines when there have been difficulties, e.g. illness that prevents proper completion of work. Do not be reluctant to negotiate an extension if you have experienced unforeseen difficulties.

Working while you are a student

Learning takes place as much from experiences gained in practice as from learning from reading, thinking and writing. As a student, you will be working as part of the course but not as an employee. Your course is unlike so many other university courses because your ultimate professional registration depends on the practical work you perform. So whereas other university students use their non-contact time (i.e. time away from lecturers) to study and socialize, much of your non-contact time is spent practising in care establishments, studying and socializing or perhaps running a household, family, etc. This means that your actual free time for yourself is limited and needs to be managed differently from the way you managed it before you started the course.

If you need to work to earn money, as discussed earlier, this will produce its own set of stresses. Taking time from social activities, study and often sleep can have effects on wakefulness, concentration and morale. Holding down a job that helps fund studies might be relatively easy at the beginning of a course but some students find that the need to concentrate on studies when the academic level increases puts a strain on their ability to work in the latter part of the course. Paid or unpaid employment reduces the time available for study. Some students seem able to compile assignments within a few weeks, others need all the time allowable and some ask for extensions to deadlines. This results in a tension between the need to earn money and the need to study; the outcome is often further stress. Disappointment can occur because assessment results are lower than anticipated or financial hardship may follow. The amount of time that is devoted to reading and reflection on, and assimilation of that reading is often related to academic results so this is another issue that is related to work time, leisure time and time off for illness.

Some students enjoy the experience of work outside their course and gain positive well-being from it. Working as a health care assistant or similar can help students gain practical experience and interactional skills. Furthermore, the experiences will help nurture a caring attitude and approach to others. However, there is a word of warning here. Some students feel compromised when they work as a bank health care assistant. They may even do such work on a ward where they have worked in the role of student nurse. Students in this situation obviously possess skills gained and practised as a student but there is a tension when they are not able to use these skills as a health care assistant. In both roles, the student is responsible to the same manager but different tasks and interactions are expected in the differing roles. Students often feel restricted when in the assistant role and should remember the boundaries to the role and the expectations made of them.

Many students continue the work that they enjoyed before starting university. Any job means that transferable skills are learned and these are very valuable to a student of nursing. Interpersonal skills, responsibility, autonomy, independence and team working are just some of them. However, some jobs are low paid and this leads to some students taking on several different jobs. A reverse situation exists because some students leave paid employment to join a course. They may lose status and other benefits of employment. The change in role, control and perceived competence can be an initial worry.

Other non-paid work may involve students using their time away from study and placement experiences to help others, in a caring role for example, or to support a partner or spouse's employment. One of my students needed to be at home to support her husband's business by performing an accountant's role; he had just become self-employed and could not afford to employ another person to help.

Reflective activity

This is a good place to encourage you to think about your commitment to others. Have a look at the following questions:

If you are currently employed, will the nature of your employment change as a result of your course?

Will you need to start a job to finance your course?

If there are people who are dependent on you for their well-being what will have to change when you start your course?

Will you be able to alter any volunteer work while on your course?

If you have any regular sporting interests, will you need to make any changes to your routines?

While thinking of the possible answers you might like to involve others in discussion to arrive at an action plan so you can control the changes that may have to be made.

Well-being is a critical factor for success

The effects on available time for study and recreation, and the effects on well-being are critical issues. However, physical manifestations of tiredness and frustration can affect behaviour and friends and associates might be the first people to recognize the results of getting the balance wrong. For this reason you may find yourself helping a friend to realize what is happening to them because the student who gets the balance wrong may not be the first to realize it.

Any physical or psychological work takes energy. A study day can be as draining, if not more

so than physical work. Routine academic study may lead to under-stimulation during the day, which may fail to induce sleep later at night. Physical work can produce more deep sleep, which can create the sense of recuperation the following day. An interesting day's activities filled with variety and novelty helps to induce sleep more rapidly and provides more deep sleep. However, extra work of any kind produces a sense of weariness after an extended time. If insomnia occurs it can lead to ill health, reduced work performance, absenteeism and accidents. If this happens, try to increase exercise and interest during the waking hours. If you are interested in sleep, a good book to read is Morgan and Closs (1999).

Students should not expect absence from work or study to be condoned and they can attract responses from placements and or the university that prove to be stressful. Each university course has regulations about minimum attendance; they might relate differently to practice and theory. These will probably be reinforced during induction. So the message is: talk to your lecturer about your need to work outside your course. Genuine sickness is usually not a cause for debate but absence levels are cause for concern during professional courses and lecturers are there to help during times of difficulty. Student welfare officers or occupational health departments can help. They can help with advice about health-related issues, counselling, finance and employment issues. Considering all these factors, there appears to be a vicious circle that could operate (Fig. 8.1).

Cause and effect of poor well-being

It is obvious that students may need support at any stage of this cycle of events to protect their well-being. Over time we build up strategies to cope with stress. McInnes (1999) comments that although these strategies might have helped in the past, that might not be the case presently in a new situation. Nursing courses help students to be more assertive and this is one skill that should help students to challenge their stressful encounters. The following is a possible **stress-relieving process** (after McInnes, 1999):

- Look at what is causing the stress and try to do what you can to alter it: you could try to tackle

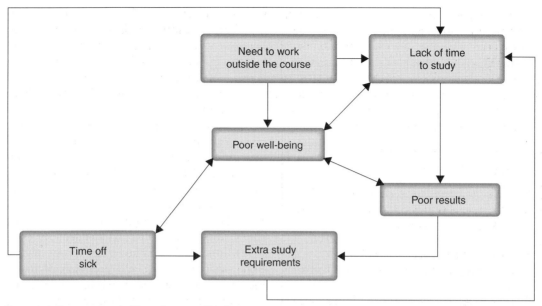

Figure 8.1 *The cause and effect of poor well-being*

bits of the problem at a time, break it down to manageable chunks.

- If that can not be done try to change your perception of it, think about trying to see it as if someone else has the problem and what they might do about it.
- Try not to worry about stress. Some stress is positive and can be a motivational force for positive change and we should not strive to erase all stress in our lives – in any case that would be impossible.

Physical and emotional changes will occur during the course. One guarantee is that at the end of the course every student will be a different person: not only because of experiences but also because maturity adds insight and a changed self-awareness. The knowledge that we as adults can be vulnerable, wrong, unskilled and unappreciated can come as a surprise. Support is often required to help explain and accept personal and attitudinal changes. Disenchantment with placements, colleagues, lecturers and results can lead to apathy, lack of motivation and does occasionally lead to students withdrawing from courses. Problems are much better aired before they affect you, let alone other people you are close to.

Illness can happen at any time, a fact that all nurses quickly learn to appreciate. A little knowledge may make you suspect the worse about personal illness. Furthermore, nursing ill people can make you think that patients' symptoms could be similar to your own. This can lead to needless worry or even hypochondriasis. Personal illness must be taken seriously, as you need to be fit and well to be able to nurse patients.

Struggling into work when ill could lead others to question your professionalism and motives. Colds and 'flu', for example, are debilitating and contagious and as such are best isolated from staff and patients, so stay at home. Occasionally courses have to be customized or interrupted because of illness. This obviously is unfortunate but not a sign of personal weakness or failure. Further advice may need to be sought regarding maximum allowable sick leave and of course, it is vital to follow any health and safety advice, policies and procedures relating to working while ill or recovering.

Reflective activity

The following exercise refers to questions that will help you to focus further on your needs for support and relate to some of the issues discussed above. If you have yet to commence a course:

What changes will occur for which you will have to make adjustments? They may be the same or similar to those identified above.

What support might you use when you are at university?

How do you think your needs for support might change when you commence a university course?

How relationships might be affected

When you start the course, it might involve an element of sacrifice, a trade of a comfortable existence for an uncertain future as borne out by Earwaker (1992). You should look to the course for re-assurance that your decision was justified. You may need to ask questions to test whether the curriculum will or will not satisfy your needs. This could be a continuous affair of challenge for you and your lecturers but during the course, you should continue this process of checking your decisions so that you re-affirm your commitment to the course and desire to succeed.

Leaving family and friends to join a course can be stressful. This of course will probably be temporary. However, for some who travel from overseas this separation might be for many months or a year or so. It is important to maintain contact because family and friends can be a tower of strong support at times when motivation decreases and they will want to know how you are progressing, especially about your successes and excitements. Try to remain in contact through any means you can, by phone, e-mail, text, letter, etc. Travelling will incur greater cost and it is probably sensible to budget wisely for trips home. As students settle down into shift patterns and blocks of study, they tend to reduce their trips home, etc. However, it should be borne in mind that homesickness can become a serious issue. You or your friends may need to help others to adjust to being away from those on whom they have significant dependence. Again, talk to tutors, friends, and welfare officers if you need to. If homesickness is a worry have a look at these websites that offer useful tips to help you through homesickness now or in the future:

- www.uwec.edu/counsel/pubs/homesick.htm
- www.counselling.cam.ac.uk/hsick.html

Family problems and home life might not be disrupted and may in fact provide substantial support (Earwaker, 1992). Some problems might even be solved by changes that the course produces. However, occasionally, changes can cause problems. Separations, financial hardship, loneliness, changes to roles or an unco-operative spouse are just a few. When the student is a lone parent and siblings require care, this can produce enormous difficulties. Childminding, escorts to and from school, planning and provision of meals, especially when shift work is involved can all be stressful. A lot of discipline may be required when trying to study at home surrounded by dependant children and spouse. Timing and time management would be essential. It would also be important to give something back to the family in the way of quality time; time that is devoted to others as their reward for the allowances they make towards you. Problems like these are surmountable and sometimes help from others is the key. Here are some suggestions (Counselling Services, 2004):

- Admit that there is a problem – talk about it with a family member or friend. Peer groups do work very well if there is a willingness to share feelings, emotions, etc. You will probably feel stronger for having shared your feelings.
- Make new friends.
- Think about what you want to gain or how you would like to change.
- Writing about your thoughts can help. When you see your ideas on paper, they can look different as if they are someone else's. You could imagine your friend has the problem, how would you advise them? Then try taking your own advice.
- Don't just complain, think what you want to change or achieve out of a situation but make your expectations achievable and realistic.
- Importantly, do something. Buried problems rear their ugly heads later when you might be less able to deal with them.

Relationships with peers are dynamic. Meeting fellow students for the first time and making and breaking ties with peers brings a different set of uncertainties, doubts or pressures. In addition, **peer pressure** still exists within groups of student nurses. For example, you may experience pressure to take up smoking or to give up smoking. Some students are enticed to join or leave groups. However, on a positive note some are encouraged to lead groups or be an official group representative. These activities might not be your initial choice, but surreptitious pressure might bring positive rewards. Remember your personal right to express your own thoughts and to make up your own mind (Townend, 1991).

It is possible to discover new interests at university. Find out details about sports activities at and around the campus. There are probably interest groups and the student union will have lots of information about their activities, which are often the centre of university life.

Most other university course students have more free time at their disposal than students of nursing. Other students may seem to be 'getting off lightly' when they seem to be out all the time or enjoying more freedom to choose whether to attend lectures. It can be frustrating if you are not expecting this. Sharing accommodation with other university students can bring a unique set of pressures. While others may be out 'clubbing', it is student nurses who have to work in placements, even during the night. Other students do not always appreciate the need for quiet and the understanding that mid-week days off replace weekends and social time might not often coincide so some mixing with others might be constrained.

Challenges for mature students

Balancing domestic responsibilities with study can be a new venture. Remember that at school or college, time had to be shared between responsibilities and to some degree you must have been successful. It has to be said that increasing age does bring with it different and often more significant responsibilities and occasionally a reduced desire to change. However, change is something that you will have committed yourself to for at least the next three years and coping with unforeseen

difficulties will probably depend on planning to cope with the known difficulties now. Good preparation is the key to a feeling of being in control and that is the key to coping so if you have doubts, ask people questions, find sources of information, listen to advice and be prepared to make difficult decisions. When difficulties are shared, they can seem to be easier to deal with. Making new friends can help in this process and remember that strangers might be simply friends that you have not yet met.

Some students need to continue to support their partner, for example, financially, emotionally, in a health care capacity or in business. This takes time, effort and commitment. It also takes understanding and tolerance from the partner. Compromises may have to be made on both sides and this might only happen after lengthy debate and heart searching. Again understanding and compromise is needed and assertiveness on both sides is a key to overall success, and the likelihood that changes will eventually change again needs to be understood so decisions will not necessarily be life-long.

For many, the challenge of re-entering education after time out causes unease. Some students have not studied for many years; they may have raised a family or for other reasons now have reduced demands from dependants. There are many reasons why some students feel that when they start a course they are in some way disadvantaged. However, mature students bring with them life experiences that others cannot possess and younger students can be very grateful for the learning that they achieve from mixing with mature students. Although the lack of recent study can be seen as a disadvantage, skills such as time management can be easily learned. The commitment to learning that mature students possess is possibly stronger than it is in some students who have just left school or college. Effective learning is often born from commitment and motivation so these should be seen as gifts that should not be underestimated.

Information and communication technology (ICT) is a part of efficient learning and certainly, the ability to use a word processor would be an advantage. Recording notes and references on a computer can easily be transformed into a presentable assignment. Time is saved which is an advantage and connection to the internet means communication with the university. Couple this with the ability to access literature on the world wide web and university libraries together with electronic journals and it is an advantage for study that should be a major consideration for students. Universities have computerized study facilities and courses include the use and teaching of ICT so a lack of experience or a perceived lack of skill will be overcome with practise.

Coping as a student from overseas

Adapting to a new place of study, new accommodation or a new town can be stressful enough but what about a new country and culture? Students may be fearful of encountering hostility or alienation from fellow students or neighbours because of where they come from, how they speak or what they look like. English might be a student's second language and it might be difficult to cope with translations and the speed of delivery of lectures. If in doubt students should seek advice to find out if there are any English-language courses run by the university. Some in fact commence before official course start dates to give students a bit of a head start. Universities usually cater for students from overseas through the operation of a support group or student support services or a dedicated overseas student office that might arrange seminars, visits or meetings.

One of the inherent difficulties faced by overseas students is the physical separation from known and trusted friends and family. The people who used to surround you are no longer near and the isolation felt can be enormous. Obviously, this can be minimized. Telephone conversations do not have to be very expensive, e-mail facilities might be useful and letters are still valued even though it is often termed 'snail mail'.

Actual visits home might be few but will be greatly valued. The possibilities, not taking into account the financial issues, must be checked well in advance as it might be very difficult to re-arrange placements and taught classes, for example, which are usually planned before you start the course. So, check for when the planned annual leave is arranged.

Summary

This section has discussed some of the common reasons why you might seek support during training. They are numerous and the list is by no means exhaustive. It is hoped that you will now imagine that although you may have many needs as a result of possible or actual changes to your lifestyle, you will, however, be able to cope. Knowing what to do about a problem is only half the battle; the other half is to do something to improve your ability to cope. Coping alone can succeed, but it might be advantageous to share experiences, because coping together with others can lead to unexpected ideas for enhancing your ability to tackle present and future challenges.

SYSTEMS OF SUPPORT DURING THE COURSE

As Phillips (1994) suggested the main thrust of support is probably of an academic nature; pastoral care is also an essential element. Most contacts initiated because of an academic need include some discussion related to the student's feelings about themselves or others. Interactions on placements, in university, conflicting demands on students' time are common discussion topics. One aim of study is to prepare students to accept responsibility for their own actions and their own learning. Learning through lectures and group sessions alone will not achieve this; personal tutorials can, through individualized advice, direction, problem-solving and reflection when they are aimed at an individual student's needs. Students will optimize the level of self-awareness if they avail themselves of this facility.

The role of personal tutor

It is not the sole province of one supporter, but the effective combination of all the available support systems available to students, that will optimize the educational experience. A lecturer who has responsibility for co-ordinating the support of students may be termed a personal tutor.

Individual students have different needs when entering university compared with their needs when leaving university, and the dynamics of the student–tutor relationship reflects this. At first, there will be a sense of dependence on the support structures in general. New relationships can be fraught with doubt and anxiety. However, try not to delay or put off meeting with a tutor. Generally, all students have an equal right to gain help from lecturers. You should try to maintain regular meetings to improve rapport, which will help you to learn more about your abilities, strengths and weaknesses. Self-awareness is a life-long process of development and it is often not possible to become aware of what others think of you unless you ask or they tell you.

Writing in a diary can help students to record their thoughts, feelings and experiences. In some courses, this can be a formal part of the curriculum. 'Reflection … is a generic term for those intellectual and affective activities in which individuals engage to explore their experiences in order to lead to new understandings and appreciations' (Boud et al., 1985 p. 19). Reflection involves thinking about all that a person does, feels and thinks about situations or events. Learning from reflection is helped in part by keeping a reflective diary or portfolio, used to recall items for discussion, during tutorials; it can be used as a very powerful tool to reflect on changes in knowledge base and importantly attitudinal changes (Heath, 1998). Reflection on action (see Schon, 1983) can contribute to growth of professional attitudes, and writing about experiences, thoughts and feelings will lead to improved self-awareness. Read also Palmer et al. (1994) to discover more about how reflection can help your professional development.

Some tutor–student relationships will be formalized. This means the tutor initiates the interactions and sets the intervals of meetings. Another approach is the very informal management of the scheme whereby students initiate meetings as and when required. This informal system often occurs alongside a more official system. The reason for this is that although students and tutors are assigned to each other, students may also have so much incidental contact with another lecturer that they decide to interact for all other support requirements with that lecturer. This should not present many problems to the organization but you may need to inform your personal tutor about how you are operating. While all concerned may not find difficulties, this could lead to some students finding their tutors unavailable due to them being in demand. Line managers may as a result rationalize the support structure and formalize the system to produce a more equitable workload among all lecturers. Phillips (1994) advocated a formally planned framework of support to be included in curricula for this reason.

Some tutors are able to organize their time to see students in a flexible manner. When students make a request, tutors may simply make an appointment in a diary to their mutual benefit. Alternatively, some tutors have so many demands on their time that they set certain times within their working week as surgery times when they would be available for students to drop in when they can. Of course, these two contrasting arrangements will not benefit all people at all times and ad hoc arrangements will always operate. Suffice to say that while it is accepted that students have a right to see their tutors, the process is dissimilar to feeling thirsty, going to a vending machine and obtaining a drink on demand. You will need to appreciate that tutors have needs, demands on their time and the need and right to coffee and lunch breaks. This should be borne in mind when knocking on a door and expecting to be seen there and then.

The variety of qualifications held by students and their individual life experiences indicate that students will experience differing levels of satisfaction from lectures and seminars. Further explanation and advice can be gained from the lecturing staff after sessions or even before sessions if they are concurrent. This of course may not occur directly after all sessions. Staff may not be available or you may be moving on to another session. For this reason you could note down the questions you have. You might like to wait for your next meeting with the lecturer but you could refer to texts on reading lists and other sources used in libraries. Your questions might also be answered by friends. The power of belief is very strong so try to believe in what you want to say or ask and do not feel reluctant to ask just because you think you might be wrong. Being a student means that you are allowed to make mistakes, often – that is how we learn.

Bramley (1977) advocated a model of friendship for the student–tutor relationship. Students should be able to expect their personal tutor to be friendly but not their best friend. If the lecturer is required to discuss poor progress or academic failure or misdemeanours with students, a personal relationship may make the exchange difficult at the least and hard for students to accept. Therefore, although you should expect a lecturer to be friendly, you should be aware that lecturers would attempt to protect you both from over-familiarity.

Friendship is not essential to the central role of support, and the personal tutor may in fact not actually teach the students. Some personal tutors may have a relationship with students for the whole of the course or for only part of it. Different institutions will have produced their list of role responsibilities from different origins. This will be demonstrated through the operation of the role.

Support by placement mentors

A network of qualified nurses and experienced staff provide support for students in placements. These nurses should be appropriately qualified and experienced in their speciality and will have attended training sessions to familiarize themselves with curricula content and assessment strategies relevant to their practice setting and course requirements. Students often say that the quality of the placement experience hinges on the quality of the relationship between them and their placement mentors. The role of the placement mentor is therefore a crucial one. Some mentors will be junior staff who have been in their role for less than a year. Relatively new mentors can be very useful to students because their training will have been recent and fresh in their mind. The stressors present for students might be identifiable by the mentor so there is a possibility of a useful empathic relationship developing.

Mentors who have many years' experience in the speciality and of supporting students are often seen as oracles of knowledge. Their confidence in approaching students and knowing how to facilitate learning through contemplation and encouraging new experiences is acknowledged by students as being invaluable and often a reason for requests to re-visit a placement at a later date.

Support in placements by lecturers

Students will also be supported in placements by lecturers who undertake key aspects of preparation. Visits will afford students the chance to discuss academic and practical developments together with discussing the theoretical underpinnings of practice. The morale of staff in placements will have an effect on your attitude and motivation. Be prepared to discuss this with your visiting lecturer who will be able to highlight issues that you may not be aware of and possibly influence the support from other people or resources during the experience. Discussions in class of course provide opportunities to explore experiences. Especially important is the need to debrief after experiences that were emotionally significant or incidents that were of a critical nature. Occasionally explanations are not given close to events and worries and questions that are left unanswered can affect morale and taint beliefs that otherwise would not be a problem. Lecturers might refer you back to practice staff but it is still important to alert lecturers to what you are experiencing either verbally or through your diary or portfolio.

Peer support

Students are a great support to each other and some believe that they only survived on a course because of their friends. Even during the preparation of assignments, it is important to share, perhaps review each other's work. Of course, several students who regularly share will be helping each other, which will be reinforcing their team spirit, and thus strengthening their confidence and group strength. This will help in the future when new challenges occur. Sometimes even competition can be very healthy as it can produce new insights and risk-taking. A group identity, though, provides security and camaraderie that is actioned often when required by an individual. For example, if a student needs to relocate accommodation, it would be friends who will probably help with the arrangements.

Help with language was mentioned earlier, and mixing with peers can be valuable as a 'safe' situation to practise speaking and reviewing their writing skills. This would provide help towards

9

Career Management and Development for Registered Nurses

Jane E Schober

INTRODUCTION

One of the most influential actions you take during your working life is making career-related decisions. Generally, choosing a job or a course of study and being selected seems achievement enough. However, making effective, relevant choices is a complex process that is central to your individual well-being and your career development. This chapter aims to offer you details and guidance relating to career management and takes into account personal, social, professional and educational factors relevant to working as a registered nurse.

The chapter is based on a **Ten Point Plan** for career development. Each point in the plan is explored in detail and serves as a framework to help you make effective career choices. The Ten Point Plan includes:

- Nursing and Midwifery Council (NMC) requirements to maintain your licence to practise nursing
- NMC requirements for returning to practice
- How to maintain your personal professional profile and your personal development plan
- Career options and opportunities available to you
- Sources of employment information
- Sources of course and educational information
- Factors affecting career choices, i.e. work needs, personal needs and family/social needs
- Factors influencing your job satisfaction
- Applying for a new job – the selection process
- How to manage the selection interview processes

NMC REQUIREMENTS TO MAINTAIN YOUR LICENCE TO PRACTISE NURSING

Becoming a registered nurse is the first step in the process of career development. It is a period filled with opportunity, challenges and excitement as professional roles are taken up in practice areas. Support and guidance is available as is the expectation from employers, professional colleagues and patients that you are able to practise safely, competently and in accordance with established standards. Post-registration education and practice (PREP) requirements and the code of professional conduct (see Appendix 2, NMC, 2002b) emphasize the need to maintain professional standards. Continuing professional development (CPD) is both a standard for achieving PREP and a process contributing to life-long learning (NMC, 2001):

> The NMC's Code of professional conduct requires you, regardless of where you are working and regardless of whether or not you are currently practising, to maintain and improve your professional knowledge and competence.

> (NMC, 2001, p. 8)

Life-long learning and continuing professional development

Nurses face many challenges during their careers and need to take responsibility for their professional development to respond effectively to changes in practice. Maintaining an enquiring approach to practice is essential to life-long learning (NMC, 2001). Keeping up to date, maintaining and developing new skills, taking advantage of learning opportunities, whether these are formal teaching sessions or informal initiatives are all part of this process. Much of this responsibility lies with the registered nurse because he or she may determine how the standards are achieved. However, the NMC PREP standards and support from employers, mentors and colleagues all contribute to the guidance and learning opportunities necessary for registered nurses (see also the section on factors influencing your job satisfaction and Chapter 8).

Renewal of registration

Nurses working in the UK are required to renew their registration every 3 years (NMC, 2002a) to practise as a nurse. This process ensures that nurses meet the standards required for registration, sign a notification of practice form and that PREP requirements are met (NMC, 2002a). Two professional standards must be met to fulfil the legal requirements for the NMC. These are:

> The PREP (practice) standard – you must have worked in some capacity by virtue of your nursing or midwifery qualification during the previous five years for a minimum of 100 days (750 hours), or have successfully undertaken an approved return to practice course.
> The PREP (continuing professional development) standard – you must have undertaken and recorded your continuing professional development (CPD) over the three years prior to the renewal of your registration. All registered nurses and midwives have been required to comply with this standard since April 1995. Since April 2000, registrants need to have declared on their NOP form that they have met this requirement when they renew their registration.

> (NMC, 2002a, p. 4)

The PREP (practice) standard

This standard may be fulfilled in a number of ways. The evidence of working as a nurse (or midwife) for

the minimum 100 days may be fulfilled by working full time, part time, voluntarily or, for example, by caring for a relative at home. If you wish to renew your nursing and midwifery registrations, 200 days would need to be completed, 100 hours for each registration.

The PREP (CPD) standard

This standard requires you to provide evidence of learning activities relevant to your practice. This is a minimum standard and should in no way discourage you from exceeding the recommended criteria which are to:

> undertake at least five days or 35 hours of learning activity relevant to your practice during the three years prior to your renewal of registration
> maintain a personal professional profile of your learning activity
> comply with any request from the NMC to audit how you have met these requirements.

> (NMC, 2002a, p. 7)

NMC REQUIREMENTS FOR RETURNING TO PRACTICE

Many nurses have a break in service during their careers. If this break is over five years long, it is an NMC requirement (Box 9.1) to attend an approved Return to Practice course to fulfil the PREP practice standard. Many centres in the UK offer these courses which are at least 5 days in length (details are available on the NHS Careers and NMC websites, see Useful websites and addresses at the end of the chapter). These courses focus on professional updating, current issues in nursing, key skills, legal

---

Box 9.1 NMC requirements for the renewal of registration

- Signed declaration that the PREP practice and CPD standards have been met
- Completed notification of practice form
- Compliance with the NMC audit
- Maintenance of a personal professional profile

issues and management of care. Successful completion of a course entitles participants to re-register with the NMC along with the notification of practice documentation and renewal fee.

HOW TO MANAGE YOUR PERSONAL PROFESSIONAL PROFILE AND YOUR PERSONAL DEVELOPMENT PLAN

Your personal professional profile is not just a requirement for PREP and CPD, it is an integral part of the educational process for pre- and post-registration learning. Many nurses have a substantial profile from their pre-registration learning courses and there may be evidence of learning from this period that is relevant to the post-registration period, particularly for those who are newly registered.

Your profile is a personal record of professional development. It is an essential record of CPD and as such should be regarded as a live document. To fulfil the PREP (CPD) requirement, the profile should contain evidence of learning activities, which may also be completed in the Welsh language. However, the profile may also include (Schober, 2003 p. 419):

- 'biographical information
- the record of qualifications, academic and professional
- a summary of current and previous posts
- details of relevant responsibilities and activities, e.g. management roles, interest groups, research activities and publications
- the record of education and formal learning experiences, e.g. courses, study days and updates, conference attendance and teaching activities
- a record of working hours during the previous 3 years
- reflection and evaluation of performance; this may also include critical incident analysis as well as examples of feedback from mentors and peers
- personal and professional objectives; this may be in the form of an action plan.'

As your profile is a PREP requirement, is has the potential to grow as a record of your nursing career (Box 9.2) and professional development. It may be used to support a job application and as a source of evidence that you may wish to refer to if working

alongside a mentor or preceptor. It may also be used to record details of experiences of nursing and caring if undertaking non-paid and voluntary work.

Box 9.2 Organizing your profile

When organizing your profile, aim to:

- keep your profile up to date
- date all entries
- structure the document logically
- use an index
- avoid names and ensure confidentiality
- keep your profile secure

Your personal development plan

As an employee and a qualified nurse, you will be entitled to support, learning opportunities and training to fulfil the requirements of your role. In the National Health Service (NHS) and in most areas of health care employment, systems of individual performance review or appraisal exist as the opportunity for your line manager to give you feedback, advice and guidance about your performance at work. These reviews usually occur at three months, six months and then annually. From this process, a personal development plan (PDP) may be referred to as an aspect of the process that confirms any learning and training needs, learning opportunities and development needs.

Your personal development plan – getting started

Your PDP may become an integral part of your personal professional profile as much information is common to them both. Planning involves reflection and self-assessment to consider your strengths, learning needs, how you will respond to the needs of the work role and the multi-professional team.

Reflective activity

Consider your current role: Do you feel confident in your abilities to fulfil the role? What are your priorities, learning needs and goals?

See Box 9.3 and compare your list with the list of skills here. Prioritize your needs and document them, these will serve as a basis for your plan and your discussion with your line manager. Consider the priorities and skills listed in Box 9.3.

Box 9.3 Examples of personal development priorities and skills

- Clinical skills
- Management skills
- Professional knowledge
- Leadership skills
- Specialist communication skills
- Academic progression
- Research skills and opportunities
- Multi-professional working methods

From the outset of your career, your PDP will help you to organize your development but without resources and support, the implementation may not be effective.

CAREER OPTIONS AND OPPORTUNITIES AVAILABLE TO YOU

Many factors affect career options and opportunities. These include your experience, qualifications, personal and social commitments which may, for example, affect your working hours and your eligibility for a post. Employment opportunities for nurses are wide ranging and there are many examples of roles which subsequently become available depending on the stage of a career (see the section on Sources of employment information).

Having chosen a branch of nursing for your pre-registration course, you have made a significant choice which gives you opportunities to discover and experience a range of options associated with that branch. This exposure to practise during a course often influences that choice of first post after registration as you may wish to return to a familiar placement, you may be invited to apply for an available post and in a few cases, you may have to return to it if you were seconded to undertake the course.

Your first post

It is not unusual for nurses who achieve their registration to apply for a first post in an NHS trust. Nurses are often encouraged to consider posts local to the higher education institution (HEI) where they undertook their course as they know the locality and associated practices. Also, this goes some way towards easing the transition from student to staff nurse which, in itself, is a complex process and it may help consolidate key skills and aspects of the course. Many students report that the uncertainty of this period is influenced by:

- concerns about impending course results
- excitement tinged with apprehension about job applications
- changes in group dynamics as course members go their own way and support networks change.

Although most nurses opt for a post in the NHS, the independent sector, e.g. private hospitals, clinics and recruitment agencies also offer posts in the UK and abroad. Key roles for newly qualified nurses (pay band 5) in the NHS are listed in Box 9.4. You

---

Box 9.4 Roles for newly qualified nurses in the NHS (pay band 5)

- Qualified nurse: adult, children's, learning disability or mental health nurse
- Community nurse
- Practice nurse
- Nurse (who works in a school)

Qualified nurses who remain in NHS employment, have a wide range of employment options as jobs are available in:

- primary, secondary and tertiary health care and practice settings
- teaching as a practice educator
- management
- research

With experience, relevant education and promotion nurses may progress from the roles of newly qualified nurses (pay band 5) to more senior NHS posts.

---

will find that there is a wide range of specialities within each branch that are shaped by the needs of the patient/client group, their dependency and the type of care required. With the development of services in the community and primary health care trusts, a wider range of roles are available for nurses from all the branches. Box 9.5 identifies key roles in the remaining pay bands for nurses in clinical practice.

SOURCES OF EMPLOYMENT INFORMATION

In addition to employment within the NHS, there is a wide range of prospective employers of nurses (Box 9.6) and because of this, you need to be mindful of the range of issues pertinent to a role. Discovering as much information as possible about a job, your employer, the parent organization and the conditions of service are vital to this process.

Box 9.5 Nurses posts and pay bands 6–8

Pay band 6
- Community psychiatric nurse
- District nurse
- Health visitor
- Deputy ward manager/ward team leader
- Nurse advisor (NHS Direct/NHS 24)
- Qualified school nurse
- Specialist nurse
- Specialist practice nurse
- Specialist theatre nurse

Pay band 7
- Ward manager
- Community psychiatric nurse manager
- Health visitor (community practice teacher)
- Highly specialist nurse
- Team manager district nursing
- Team manager health visiting
- Team manager school nursing
- Sexual health advisory service manager (community)

Pay band 8
- Consultant nurse – range A and B
- Professional manager – range C and D

Box 9.6 Employers of nurses in the UK

- Charitable organizations, e.g. Macmillan nurses
- HM forces, e.g. army, navy and air force
- HEIs/universities
- Nursing agencies
- Overseas development services, e.g. the British Red Cross
- Independent health care organizations
- Pharmaceutical companies
- Professional organizations, e.g. the Royal College of Nursing
- Statutory organizations
- Trade unions

Initially finding a job is a central goal, particularly at the end of a course or following a period of leave or travel. Prospective employees tend to refer to specialist journals, local and national press for details of available posts. Box 9.7 lists additional sources of employment information that highlight how to access information about available jobs and where to gain information about an employer.

Box 9.7 Other sources of employment information

- Human resources departments within organizations
- Internal communications, e.g. newsletters
- Parent organization websites, e.g. local NHS trust

Details of NHS posts and qualifications required for these posts are available on the NHS and NMC websites (see Useful websites). Details specific to each country in the UK are also available (see Useful addresses and websites).

In addition, you need to be confident about what a prospective employer is able to offer you. The elements of employment which may affect your decision to apply include:

- employment policies, i.e. how policies are operationalized, e.g. family-friendly policies, staff development
- terms and conditions of service, e.g. contract, salary and leave details
- staff support networks, e.g. preceptorship scheme, mentor support, personal development planning and individual performance review (IPR)
- quality assurance mechanisms
- induction programme and staff training.

Job advertisements usually provide summary information about a job and the employer. When applying for a post exploring this employer-specific information is vital. In the section on How to manage the selection interview processes, the issues relating to applying for a job and the selection process are explored further.

Working abroad

Many nurses use their professional qualifications to travel and work abroad. There is a range of employment agencies, charities and overseas development organizations that co-ordinate this. Most countries have requirements for employment and professional registration. The European Union (EU) has legislation that facilitates the employment of nurses registered in the UK. To nurse abroad you should be conversant with:

- registration requirements
- employment conditions, contract details and accommodation
- visa and work permit requirements
- indemnity and medical insurance options
- tax, pensions and leave entitlements
- personal health issues
- language issues.

Some countries, e.g. USA, require nurses to pass exams before they will consider their employment. Usually these are completed in the UK. Details of such requirements may be accessed through international nursing and health care recruitment agencies (see Useful addresses).

Applying to nurse abroad is a complex and often time-consuming process. It is always advisable to seek advice from reputable sources, e.g. the Royal College of Nursing (RCN) International office and the NMC (see Useful addresses).

Sources of course and educational information

The diversity of nursing and health care, the rates of change in practice, policy and roles and professional recommendations for ongoing education make it essential for nurses to adopt strategies for life-long learning. Identifying what is available, what is accessible and what is relevant and necessary is a complex business. Here, therefore, is an outline of resources which will support this process of ongoing learning.

General career and course information

By visiting the NHS career and NMC websites you will access general information about key roles and their educational requirements. In addition each UK country has its own website for nurses that offer the latest details about professional development and courses (see Useful addresses).

Career advice and guidance – the case for a mentor

Finding out about educational opportunities is part of the wider life-long learning and CPD process. As such, it is necessary to discover the opportunities available as well as having advice to assist decisions. Career advice is rarely a formal part of an employee's support network, rather, it is usually integral to relationships which emerge at work. This is particularly true of relationships between nurses and their line managers, as senior colleagues may have knowledge of local and national opportunities, hence the relationship with CPD.

It is not unusual for employees to initiate systems for mentoring staff. Indeed, student nurses are familiar with mentorship from their pre-registration courses. Whether this is a formal requirement or an informal system of support, a mentor relationship may develop as a catalyst for CPD and career development. This places enormous responsibility on the mentor to provide appropriate support, guidance and advice. Though mentors may have a good working knowledge of local and speciality-based career details, it is usually necessary to access other sources of information to ensure relevant information is available.

Continuing professional development

Key aspects of CPD and personal development planning depend on the availability of resources for learning. Within the NHS, there is emphasis on work-based and team learning (Department of Health (DoH), 2001) as a means of co-ordinating education and skill development. Multi-professional learning facilitates the sharing of learning opportunities and resources between professional groups and is particularly effective in relation to, for example, communication skills development, medicolegal issues and practice updates. Many local courses, whether they be short study days or longer courses, are accredited with academic credits and validated by an HEI. This is usually a feature of learning modules which are part of a longer course. This system allows credit for learning to be awarded following successful completion. It is also more flexible as most of these courses are part time and may run more than once per annum.

Higher education institutions, universities

Higher education institutions work in close partnership with a range of employers including NHS trusts and the independent health care sector. This relationship has resulted in the development of courses and learning opportunities which are central to the CPD of nurses and the support for specialist courses, e.g. specialist nurses, district nurses, health visitors and nurse teachers, as well as role developments, e.g. nurse prescribing. The HEIs' websites and prospectus will summarize the courses on offer. This information is vital for choosing a relevant course, negotiating study leave and applying for any available resources to cover course fees and required mentor support.

Open and distant learning

Open and distant learning opportunities are a flexible option for many nurses who choose to fit a course of study around their lifestyle needs. In recent years this flexibility has developed further through e-learning and this is a popular facility in HEIs. You may find that certain modules within a taught course may be studied in this way, the HEI prospectus and course information will clarify these options.

Royal College of Nursing study hours

The RCN offers a scheme for accrediting learning through the CPD article published regularly in the *Nursing Standard*. Not only does this strategy encourage professional learning, it can be used as evidence for PREP and become part of your portfolio.

Other courses

There is a wide range of topics and subjects on offer through CPD programmes and other courses. Also the academic level of courses may vary in complexity usually from diploma level, through to first degree, master's level and ultimately PhD. In general, those working at the level of pay band 5 will have achieved a diploma or first degree as part of their pre-registration course. Subsequently, roles for pay bands 6–8 would necessitate further study at first degree level. Nurse consultants and nurse teachers in HEIs would need to have undertaken study at master's level for eligibility for most posts at this level.

FACTORS AFFECTING CAREER CHOICES

Awareness has grown among employees and employers of factors that encourage commitment and well-being at work. These needs are summarized in Box 9.8 (from Schober, 1990, who identifies factors that you may find relevant to career development decisions). Consider these alongside previously detailed employment, professional and educational perspectives.

Box 9.8 Factors affecting career choices

- Work needs
- Need to work
- Promotion

- Motivation and opportunities to learn and develop professionally
- Interest/commitment to the work and role
- Range of responsibility
- Dynamics of the team and management structure
- Personal needs
- Job satisfaction
- Job security
- Status of the role
- Salary
- Reluctance to change roles
- Terms of the contract
- Family/social needs
- Family need for income
- Childcare availability
- Availability of accommodation
- Travelling distance from home
- House prices
- Support of partner/family members

Source: Schober (1990)

Reflective activity

Consider this list (Box 9.8) when assessing a new job. Prioritize the factors important to your personal, professional and social life to ascertain to what extent your new job will fulfil your needs. If you are prepared to compromise, can you anticipate short- or long-term outcomes?

Be aware of any compromise that may impact on your job satisfaction as this is a vital motivator.

FACTORS INFLUENCING YOUR JOB SATISFACTION

Job satisfaction remains the central tenet to employees remaining committed and loyal to a work role and those associated with it. Lack of job satisfaction, by implication, results in higher staff turnover and low morale. Although pay is an important factor for us all, and despite the ongoing debates about pay levels, the influence on job satisfaction is nebulous. Pay becomes more significant when employees face the demands of high-cost accommodation, travel and living expenses, particularly in south-east England and in cities.

Job satisfaction is mainly influenced in clinical posts by effective support networks e.g. preceptorship, mentoring and teamwork. Leadership styles that promote staff well-being, professional development and overall commitment to the client or patient group requiring care, are also essential.

Summary

Managing your career development depends on:

- assessment of employment opportunities
- assessment of work, personal and social needs
- information retrieval about options, the job and educational opportunities
- personal and professional support and mentorship
- fulfilment of PREP and CPD requirements
- maximizing personal and professional development opportunities.

APPLYING FOR A NEW JOB: THE SELECTION PROCESS

Having explored the factors affecting career development, they may now be used to positively influence job applications and the selection process. Your awareness of the jobs appropriate to your needs, and how relevant your skills and expertise are for an available job, are necessary prerequisites.

Finding a job

Earlier in the chapter employment opportunities for nurses were considered. Adverts for jobs are the best means of finding a job but the detail given may be very variable. Subscribing to a relevant professional journal and using the internet are vital sources for advertisements. Details of a job may then be sent for which should provide you with key information. Aim to have information that clarifies details of:

- location of the post
- contract details, grade and pay band

- role description
- term and conditions of employment
- prerequisites, e.g. qualifications and required experience
- opportunities for support and staff development
- IPR/appraisal scheme
- closing date for applications.

Elements of preparing an application

The informal visit

If you are applying for a job in a new location, an informal visit is invaluable. This gives you the opportunity to visit the place of work, meet staff, assess the environment and observe, though briefly, aspects of practice. Some employees may not facilitate such a visit, but others will and realize that you are taking your application seriously. A visit may mark whether to pursue an application or not.

Completing the application form

Any application must be accurate and beautifully presented. Remember, it is usually photocopied for all the members of an interview panel so black ink is essential. Ensure that where necessary, any requests for details relating to your motives for the application are written objectively to highlight your skills, relevance of your experience, your interest in the job and what qualities you are offering. You may find it helpful to use the sub-headings on the role description to help you organize this section.

The health assessment form

Usually a health assessment form is requested as part of the application process. This is sent directly to the occupational health department who will advise you if further details are required.

Previous convictions

Previous convictions must be declared on request and your police record will be checked if you work with vulnerable people.

Your referees

It is usual for the names of two referees to be requested. If this is a job following qualification, your HEI will be approached for a reference. Otherwise referees will be approached for a comprehensive analysis of your suitability for the post.

Choose your referees carefully, they are advocates and supporters of your professional development. You need to choose them on the basis of their understanding of your skills, qualities, career aspirations and commitment. They should know you well, perhaps they have been your manager or lecturer. Liaise with them over all your career moves so that they remain fully conversant with your plans. Give feedback following a selection process, whatever the outcome.

Your curriculum vitae

It is usual for a curriculum vitae (CV) to accompany an application form, particularly if this is a post beyond pay band 5. A CV is a support document and should provide complementary and additional information to that on the application form. Adapt key aspects of your CV to the post you are applying for. This will strengthen your application further. The CV should not replace an application form unless the application is by CV only. There is no standard format for a CV, and Box 9.9 provides a suggested outline.

Box 9.9 Developing your CV

A CV should include your:

- Name
- Address
- Contact phone/e-mail
- PIN number
- Qualifications
- Previous experience
- Professional activities

Reflective activity

If you have not already done so, prepare your CV. It may be kept with your professional profile and be updated according to any job application you make. In addition to the outline given (Box 9.9), you may wish to include details of other employment, information relating to gaps in employment and any voluntary work you undertake.

HOW TO MANAGE THE SELECTION INTERVIEW PROCESSES

A range of selection procedures may be used for selecting a candidate for a job. The method and complexity of the process will depend on the seniority of the post. For most clinical nursing jobs, the panel interview is the most popular. It follows the receipt of application papers and any short-listing procedures that ensure the criteria for the job have been met by each candidate.

Being called for interview

Notification will give you time for final preparation. Most candidates feel apprehensive prior to the event so thorough preparation is vital. This may include:

- thorough revision of your application form and CV as they relate to the criteria for the post
- revision of key professional and clinical issues as they relate to the post
- consideration of your key strengths and motives for applying
- details of how you keep up to date and fulfil PREP requirements
- preparing questions to ask at interview to clarify any key points
- planning for the day of interview including appropriate dress and travel arrangements.

The presentation

Some selection procedures require candidates to give a presentation on a given topic. This requires preparation of slides or a computer presentation such as in PowerPoint (Microsoft) for a high standard to be achieved. Hard copies of the content may be prepared for those receiving the presentation.

The interview

Panel interviews usually consist of two or more members. They may include the line manager, a senior manager, an educationalist and a member of the human resources team. Questions will relate to the application, the criteria for the post, professional awareness, key skills and team working. In addition, you may be asked to respond to a problem-based question relating to practice, issues associated with

your teaching and management skills and your career aspirations. The interview is your opportunity to communicate your skills, potential and suitability for the job. It is also a time to demonstrate your commitment, enthusiasm and professionalism.

Summary

Professional and career development depends on:

- fulfilling CPD and PREP requirements
- maintaining your PDP
- using support networks for ongoing development
- thorough assessment of career and educational opportunities
- thorough planning for all application and selection interviews
- commitment to life-long learning.

CONCLUSION

This chapter has explored key issues necessary for career and professional development. Nurses are charged with the responsibility for maintaining their licence to practice nursing as well as being competent accountable practitioners. This chapter will support you in this process.

REFERENCES

Department of Health (2001) *Working Together, Learning Together: a framework for lifelong learning for the NHS.* London: DoH.

Nursing and Midwifery Council (2001) *Supporting Nurses and Midwives through Lifelong Learning.* London: NMC.

Nursing and Midwifery Council (2002a) *The PREP Handbook.* London: NMC.

Nursing and Midwifery Council (2002b) *The NMC Code of Professional Conduct: standards for conduct, performance and ethics.* London: NMC.

Schober JE (1990) Your career – making the choices. In: Tschudin V, Schober JE (eds) *Managing Yourself.* London: Macmillan.

Schober JE (2003) Maintaining a licence to practice: your career as a professional nurse. In: Hinchliff S, Norman SE, Schober JE (eds) *Nursing Practice and Health Care*, 4th edn. London: Arnold.

ANNOTATED FURTHER READING

Hinchliff S, Norman SE, Schober JE (eds) (2003) *Nursing Practice and Health Care*, 4th edn. London: Arnold. A comprehensive textbook for all nurses studying nursing and for those returning to nursing. This multi-authored text provides the reader with a wide range of professional and practice-based issues including ethical and professional issues, working in a health care team, delivering care to a range of patient/client groups and developments in nurses' roles.

Nursing and Midwifery Council (2002) *The PREP Handbook*. London: NMC. This vital publication is essential for all nurses. It confirms the statutory requirements for re-registration and returning to nursing.

Ryder T (2000) *Health Professionals Abroad. A Directory of Worldwide Opportunities*. Oxford: Vacation Work. A useful guide to working overseas in a range of health care settings. It refers to opportunities in state and private sectors and offers practical advice about work permits, conditions of service, etc. Some of these details would need checking for any recent changes.

USEFUL WEBSITES

www.myworkplace.nhs.uk – a website to assist NHS nurses to gain as much as possible from the internet.

www.nursingintheuk.co.uk – a site for advice for nurses who trained outside the UK and who wish to work in the UK.

www.jobs.nhs.uk/ – a website listing job vacancies in the NHS including return to nursing information.

www.nhsplus.nhs.uk – a website relating to occupational health.

USEFUL ADDRESSES

Careers advice for applicants to pre-registration nursing courses

England
NHS Careers
PO Box 376
Bristol BS99 3EY
Tel: 0845 60 60 655 – Careers Helpline
www.nhscareers.nhs.com

Scotland
NHS Education for Scotland, Careers Information Service
22 Queen Street
Edinburgh EH2 1NT
www.nes.scot.nhs.uk

Wales
Health Provisions Wales
www.hpw.org.uk

Learn Direct
Tel: 0900 100900

Northern Ireland
Northern Ireland Practice and Education Council for Nursing
www.nipec.n-i.nhs.uk

Organizations offering advice for applicants to pre-registration nursing courses

Degree courses
Universities and Colleges Admissions Service (UCAS)
Rosehill
New Barn Lane
Cheltenham
Gloucestershire GL52 3LZ
Tel: 0870 112 2200 (Applications)
Tel: 0870 112 2211 (General enquiries)
www.ucas.ac.uk

Diploma courses
England
Nursing and Midwifery Admissions Service (NMAS)
Rosehill
New Barn Lane
Cheltenham
Gloucestershire GL52 3LZ
Tel: 0870 112 2200 (Applications package)
Tel: 0870 112 2206 (General enquiries)
www.nmas.ac.uk

Scotland
NBS Catch
PO Box 21
Edinburgh EH2 1NT
Tel: 0131 247 6622 (Applications)
www.nes.scot.nhs.uk

Northern Ireland

Careers advice
School of Nursing and Midwifery
Registry Office
Queen's University of Belfast
1–3 College Park East
Belfast BT7 1LQ
Tel: 028 9027 2233

Wales

Learn Direct
Tel: 0800 100 900

Professional and regulatory bodies related to nursing, midwifery and health visiting

Nursing and Midwifery Council (NMC)
23 Portland Place
London
Tel: 020 7637 7181
www.nmc-uk.org

NMC Registration Department

United Kingdom registration: Tel: 020 7333 9333
Overseas registration Tel: 020 7333 9333
Outside EU enquiries: Tel: 020 7333 6600
Professional advice: Tel: 020 7333 6541/6550/6553
Professional Conduct: Tel: 020 7333 6564
Finance: Tel: 020 7333 6652

British Association of Counselling (BAC)
1 Regent Place
Rugby
Warwickshire CV21 2PJ
Tel: 01788 550 899
www.counselling.co.uk

Community Practitioners' and Health Visitors' Association
40 Bermondsey Street
London SE1 3UD
Tel: 0207 939 7000
www.msfcphva.org

Department of Health (Publications)
PO Box 777
London SE1 6XH
E-mail: doh@prolog.uk.com
www.dh.gov.uk/Home/fs/en

Institute of Psychiatry
16 De Crespigny Park
London SE5 8AF
Tel: 020 7703 5411

The King's Fund
11–13 Cavendish Square
London W1G OAN
Tel: 020 7307 2400
www. kingsfund.org.uk

Royal College of Midwives
15 Mansfield Street
London W1G 9NH
Tel: 020 7312 3535
www. rcm.org.uk

Royal College of Nursing
20 Cavendish Square
London W1M 0AB
Tel: 020 7409 3333
www.rcn.org.uk
www.rcn.org.uk/resources/becomenurse.php

RCN Direct
Tel: 08457 726100 (24-hour advice line for
    members)
RCN Nurseline
Tel: 020 7647 3463 (10 am to 4 pm Monday to
    Friday)
RCN Counselling Service
Tel: 0845 769 7064

UNISON
1 Mabledon Place
London WC1H 9AJ
Tel: 020 7388 2366

Working Injured Nurses Group (WING)
Tel: 020 7647 3465

Financial support and student grants

NHS Student Grants
Department of Health
PO Box 777
London SE1 6XH
Tel: 08701 555 455
www.dh.gov.uk/Home/fs/en

Immigration and Nationality Directorate
The Home Office
Lunar House
40 Wellesley Road
Croydon
CR9 2BY
Tel: 020 8686 0688

NHS Pensions Agency
200–220 Broadway
Fleetwood
Lancashire FY7 8LG

Working abroad

Nursing Abroad
PO Box 8
Bakewell
Derbyshire DE45 1YG
Tel: 01629 640980
www.nursingabroad.net
www.raleighinternational.org

Appendices

Standard 7 – First level nurses – nursing standards of education to achieve the NMC standards of proficiency

Standard of proficiency for entry to the register: professional and ethical practice

Manage oneself, one's practice, and that of others, in accordance with *The NMC code of professional conduct: standards for conduct, performance and ethics*, recognising one's own abilities and limitations

Domain	Outcomes to be achieved for entry to the branch programme	Standards of proficiency for entry to the register: professional and ethical practice
Professional and ethical practice	*Discuss in an informed manner the implications of professional regulation for nursing practice* • demonstrate a basic knowledge of professional regulation and self-regulation • recognise and acknowledge the limitations of one's own abilities • recognise situations that require referral to a registered practitioner. *Demonstrate an awareness of The NMC code of professional conduct: standards for conduct, performance and ethics* • commit to the principle that the primary purpose of the registered nurse is to protect and serve society • accept responsibility for one's own actions and decisions.	• practise in accordance with *The NMC code of professional conduct: standards for conduct, performance and ethics* • use professional standards of practice to self-assess performance • consult with a registered nurse when nursing care requires expertise beyond one's own current scope of competence • consult other health care professionals when individual or group needs fall outside the scope of nursing practice • identify unsafe practice and respond appropriately to ensure a safe outcome • manage the delivery of care services within the sphere of one's own accountability.

Standard of proficiency for entry to the register: professional and ethical practice

Practise in accordance with an ethical and legal framework which ensures the primacy of patient and client interest and well-being and respects confidentiality

Domain	Outcomes to be achieved for entry to the branch programme	Standards of proficiency for entry to the register: professional and ethical practice
Professional and ethical practice	*Demonstrate an awareness of, and apply ethical principles to, nursing practice* • demonstrate respect for patient and client confidentiality • identify ethical issues in day to day practice. *Demonstrate an awareness of legislation relevant to nursing practice* • identify key issues in relevant legislation relating to mental health, children, data protection, manual handling, and health and safety, etc.	• demonstrate knowledge of legislation and health and social policy relevant to nursing practice • ensure the confidentiality and security of written and verbal information acquired in a professional capacity • demonstrate knowledge of contemporary ethical issues and their impact on nursing and health care • manage the complexities arising from ethical and legal dilemmas • act appropriately when seeking access to caring for patients and clients in their own homes.

Standard of proficiency for entry to the register: professional and ethical practice

Practise in a fair and anti-discriminatory way, acknowledging the differences in beliefs and cultural practices of individuals or groups

Domain	Outcomes to be achieved for entry to the branch programme	Standards of proficiency for entry to the register: professional and ethical practice
Professional and ethical practice	*Demonstrate the importance of promoting equity in patient and client care by contributing to nursing care in a fair and anti-discriminatory way* • demonstrate fairness and sensitivity when responding to patients, clients and groups from diverse circumstances • recognise the needs of patients and clients whose lives are affected by disability, however manifest.	• maintain, support and acknowledge the rights of individuals or groups in the health care setting • act to ensure that the rights of individuals and groups are not compromised • respect the values, customs and beliefs of individuals and groups • provide care which demonstrates sensitivity to the diversity of patients and clients.

Standard of proficiency for entry to the register: care delivery

Engage in, develop and disengage from therapeutic relationships through the use of appropriate communication and interpersonal skills

Domain	Outcomes to be achieved for entry to the branch programme	Standards of proficiency for entry to the register: care delivery
Care delivery	*Discuss methods of, barriers to, and the boundaries of, effective communication and interpersonal relationships*	• utilise a range of effective and appropriate communication and engagement skills

Domain	Outcomes to be achieved for entry to the branch programme	Standards of proficiency for entry to the register: care delivery
	• recognise the effect of one's own values on interactions with patients and clients and their carers, families and friends • utilise appropriate communication skills with patients and clients • acknowledge the boundaries of a professional caring relationship. *Demonstrate sensitivity when interacting with and providing information to patients and clients.*	• maintain and, where appropriate, disengage from professional caring relationships that focus on meeting the patient's or client's needs within professional therapeutic boundaries.

Standard of proficiency for entry to the register: care delivery

Create and utilise opportunities to promote the health and well-being of patients, clients and groups

Domain	Outcomes to be achieved for entry to the branch programme	Standards of proficiency for entry to the register: care delivery
Care delivery	*Contribute to enhancing the health and social well-being of patients and clients by understanding how, under the supervision of a registered practitioner, to:* • *contribute to the assessment of health needs* • *identify opportunities for health promotion* • *identify networks of health and social care services.*	• consult with patients, clients and groups to identify their need and desire for health promotion advice • provide relevant and current health information to patients, clients and groups in a form which facilitates their understanding and acknowledges choice/individual preference • provide support and education in the development and/or maintenance of independent living skills • seek specialist/expert advice as appropriate.

Standard of proficiency for entry to the register: care delivery

Undertake and document a comprehensive, systematic and accurate nursing assessment of the physical, psychological, social and spiritual needs of patients, clients and communities

Domain	Outcomes to be achieved for entry to the branch programme	Standards of proficiency for entry to the register: care delivery
Care delivery	*Contribute to the development and documentation of nursing assessments by participating in comprehensive and systematic nursing assessment of the physical, psychological, social and spiritual needs of patients and clients* • *be aware of assessment strategies to guide the collection of data for assessing patients and clients and use assessment tools under guidance* • *discuss the prioritisation of care needs* • *be aware of the need to reassess patients and clients as to their needs for nursing care.*	• select valid and reliable assessment tools for the required purpose • systematically collect data regarding the health and functional status of individuals, clients and communities through appropriate interaction, observation and measurement • analyse and interpret data accurately to inform nursing care and take appropriate action.

Standard of proficiency for entry to the register: care delivery

Formulate and document a plan of nursing care, where possible, in partnership with patients, clients, their carers and family and friends, within a framework of informed consent

Domain	Outcomes to be achieved for entry to the branch programme	Standards of proficiency for entry to the register: care delivery
Care delivery	*Contribute to the planning of nursing care, involving patients and clients and, where possible, their carers; demonstrating an understanding of helping patients and clients to make informed decisions* • identify care needs based on the assessment of a patient or client • participate in the negotiation and agreement of the care plan with the patient or client and with their carer, family or friends, as appropriate, under the supervision of a registered nurse • inform patients and clients about intended nursing actions, respecting their right to participate in decisions about their care.	• establish priorities for care based on individual or group needs • develop and document a care plan to achieve optimal health, habilitation, and rehabilitation based on assessment and current nursing knowledge • identify expected outcomes, including a time frame for achievement and/or review in consultation with patients, clients, their carers and family and friends and with members of the health and social care team.

Standard of proficiency for entry to the register: care delivery

Based on the best available evidence, apply knowledge and an appropriate repertoire of skills indicative of safe and effective nursing practice

Domain	Outcomes to be achieved for entry to the branch programme	Standards of proficiency for entry to the register: care delivery
Care delivery	*Contribute to the implementation of a programme of nursing care, designed and supervised by registered practitioners* • undertake activities that are consistent with the care plan and within the limits of one's own abilities. *Demonstrate evidence of a developing knowledge base which underpins safe and effective nursing practice* • access and discuss research and other evidence in nursing and related disciplines • identify examples of the use of evidence in planned nursing interventions. *Demonstrate a range of essential nursing skills, under the supervision of a registered nurse, to meet individuals' needs, which include:* maintaining dignity, privacy and confidentiality; effective communication and observational skills, including listening and taking physiological measurements; safety and health, including moving, and handling and infection control; essential first aid and emergency procedures; administration of medicines; emotional, physical and personal care, including meeting the need for comfort, nutrition and personal hygiene.	• ensure that current research findings and other evidence are incorporated in practice • identify relevant changes in practice or new information and disseminate it to colleagues • contribute to the application of a range of interventions which support and optimise the health and well-being of patients and clients • demonstrate the safe application of the skills required to meet the needs of patients and clients within the current sphere of practice • identify and respond to patients and clients' continuing learning and care needs • engage with, and evaluate, the evidence base that underpins safe nursing practice.

Standard of proficiency for entry to the register: care delivery

Provide a rationale for the nursing care delivered which takes account of social, cultural, spiritual, legal, political and economic influences

Domain	Outcomes to be achieved for entry to the branch programme	Standards of proficiency for entry to the register: care delivery
Care delivery		• identify, collect and evaluate information to justify the effective utilisation of resources to achieve planned outcomes of nursing care.

Standard of proficiency for entry to the register: care delivery

Evaluate and document the outcomes of nursing and other interventions

Domain	Outcomes to be achieved for entry to the branch programme	Standards of proficiency for entry to the register: care delivery
Care delivery	*Contribute to the evaluation of the appropriateness of nursing care delivered* • demonstrate an awareness of the need to assess regularly a patient's or client's response to nursing interventions • provide for a supervising registered practitioner, evaluative commentary and information on nursing care based on personal observations and actions • contribute to the documentation of the outcomes of nursing interventions.	• collaborate with patients and clients and, when appropriate, additional carers to review and monitor the progress of individuals or groups towards planned outcomes • analyse and revise expected outcomes, nursing interventions and priorities in accordance with changes in the individual's condition, needs or circumstances.

Standard of proficiency for entry to the register: care delivery

Demonstrate sound clinical judgement across a range of differing professional and care delivery contexts

Domain	Outcomes to be achieved for entry to the branch programme	Standards of proficiency for entry to the register: care delivery
Care delivery	*Recognise situations in which agreed plans of nursing care no longer appear appropriate and refer these to an appropriate accountable practitioner* • demonstrate the ability to discuss and accept care decisions • accurately record observations made and communicate these to the relevant members of the health and social care team.	• use evidence based knowledge from nursing and related disciplines to select and individualise nursing interventions • demonstrate the ability to transfer skills and knowledge to a variety of circumstances and settings • recognise the need for adaptation and adapt nursing practice to meet varying and unpredictable circumstances • ensure that practice does not compromise the nurse's duty of care to individuals or the safety of the public.

Standard of proficiency for entry to the register: care management

Contribute to public protection by creating and maintaining a safe environment of care through the use of quality assurance and risk management strategies

Domain	Outcomes to be achieved for entry to the branch programme	Standards of proficiency for entry to the register: care management
Care management	*Contribute to the identification of actual and potential risks to patients, clients and their carers, to oneself and to others, and participate in measures to promote and ensure health and safety* • *understand and implement health and safety principles and policies* • *recognise and report situations that are potentially unsafe for patients, clients, oneself and others.*	• apply relevant principles to ensure the safe administration of therapeutic substances • use appropriate risk assessment tools to identify actual and potential risks • identify environmental hazards and eliminate and/or prevent where possible • communicate safety concerns to a relevant authority • manage risk to provide care which best meets the needs and interests of patients, clients and the public.

Standard of proficiency for entry to the register: care management

Demonstrate knowledge of effective inter-professional working practices which respect and utilise the contributions of members of the health and social care team

Domain	Outcomes to be achieved for entry to the branch programme	Standards of proficiency for entry to the register: care management
Care management	*Demonstrate an understanding of the role of others by participating in inter-professional working practice* • *identify the roles of the members of the health and social care team* • *work within the health and social care team to maintain and enhance integrated care.*	• establish and maintain collaborative working relationships with members of the health and social care team and others • participate with members of the health and social care team in decision-making concerning patients and clients • review and evaluate care with members of the health and social care team and others.

Standard of proficiency for entry to the register: care management

Delegate duties to others, as appropriate, ensuring that they are supervised and monitored

Domain	Outcomes to be achieved for entry to the branch programme	Standards of proficiency for entry to the register: care management
Care management		• take into account the role and competence of staff when delegating work • maintain one's own accountability and responsibility when delegating aspects of care to others • demonstrate the ability to co-ordinate the delivery of nursing and health care.

Standard of proficiency for entry to the register: care management

Demonstrate key skills

Domain	Outcomes to be achieved for entry to the branch programme	Standards of proficiency for entry to the register: care management
Care management	*Demonstrate literacy, numeracy and computer skills needed to record, enter, store, retrieve and organise data essential for care delivery*	<ul><li>literacy – interpret and present information in a comprehensible manner</li><li>numeracy – accurately interpret numerical data and their significance for the safe delivery of care</li><li>information technology and management – interpret and utilise data and technology, taking account of legal, ethical and safety considerations, in the delivery and enhancement of care</li><li>problem-solving – demonstrate sound clinical decision-making which can be justified even when made on the basis of limited information.</li></ul>

Standard of proficiency for entry to the register: personal and professional development

Demonstrate a commitment to the need for continuing professional development and personal supervision activities in order to enhance knowledge, skills, values and attitudes needed for safe and effective nursing practice

Domain	Outcomes to be achieved for entry to the branch programme	Standards of proficiency for entry to the register: personal and professional development
Personal and professional development	*Demonstrate responsibility for one's own learning through the development of a portfolio of practice and recognise when further learning is required*<ul><li>*identify specific learning needs and objectives*</li><li>*begin to engage with, and interpret, the evidence base which underpins nursing practice.*</li></ul>*Acknowledge the importance of seeking supervision to develop safe and effective nursing practice*	<ul><li>identify one's own professional development needs by engaging in activities such as reflection in, and on, practice and lifelong learning</li><li>develop a personal development plan which takes into account personal, professional and organisational needs</li><li>share experiences with colleagues and patients and clients in order to identify the additional knowledge and skills needed to manage unfamiliar or professionally challenging situations</li><li>take action to meet any identified knowledge and skills deficit likely to affect the delivery of care within the current sphere of practice.</li></ul>

Standard of proficiency for entry to the register: personal and professional development

Enhance the professional development and safe practice of others through peer support, leadership, supervision and teaching

Domain	Outcomes to be achieved for entry to the branch programme	Standards of proficiency for entry to the register: personal and professional development
Personal and professional development		• contribute to creating a climate conducive to learning • contribute to the learning experiences and development of others by facilitating the mutual sharing of knowledge and experience • demonstrate effective leadership in the establishment and maintenance of safe nursing practise.

ACCESS TO THE REGISTER BY EUROPEAN SECOND LEVEL NURSES

Second level nurses trained in a European Economic Area [EEA] country are eligible to apply for entry to the NMC register. Those who wish to work in the UK must first apply to the registering body (competent authority) in their own country who will confirm their eligibility under European Law to work in the UK. They may then apply to the NMC providing copies of their certificates, confirmation of good health and good character, verification in accordance with EU Directives, photocopy of passport or identity card and Register extract where appropriate. Nurses who are registered in another EEA State but who are not nationals of an EEA State will be treated as overseas applicants, taking into account that they have been registered in another EEA State.

Such nurses who register with the NMC will be deemed to have met the standards of proficiency for second level nurses. Once registered, they will have the right to access continuing professional development to advance their knowledge, skills and proficiency beyond that of initial registration. They may also enter a pre-registration nursing programme to enable them to become a first level nurse. They may seek appropriate accreditation of prior learning, in accordance with NMC nursing standards 3 and 4, to enable them to undertake a shortened programme of preparation.

The NMC Code of Professional Conduct: standards for conduct, performance and ethics
Protecting the public through professional standards

The *Code of professional conduct* was published by the Nursing and Midwifery Council in April 2002 and came into effect on 1 June 2002. In August 2004 an addendum was published and the *Code of professional conduct* had its name changed to *The NMC code of professional conduct: standards for conduct, performance and ethics*. All references to "nurses, midwives and health visitors" were replaced by "nurses, midwives and specialist community public health nurses" and a new section on Indemnity Insurance was included. This updated version of the code was published in November 2004.

The NMC code of professional conduct: standards for conduct, performance and ethics

As a registered nurse, midwife or specialist community public health nurse, you are personally accountable for your practice. In caring for patients and clients, you must:

- respect the patient or client as an individual
- obtain consent before you give any treatment or care
- protect confidential information
- co-operate with others in the team
- maintain your professional knowledge and competence
- be trustworthy
- act to identify and minimise risk to patients and clients.

These are the shared values of all the United Kingdom health care regulatory bodies.

---

1 Introduction

1.1 The purpose of *The NMC code of professional conduct: standards for conduct, performance and ethics* is to:
- inform the professions of the standard of professional conduct required of them in the exercise of their professional accountability and practice

- inform the public, other professions and employers of the standard of professional conduct that they can expect of a registered practitioner.

1.2   As a registered nurse, midwife or specialist community public health nurse, you must:
- protect and support the health of individual patients and clients
- protect and support the health of the wider community
- act in such a way that justifies the trust and confidence the public have in you
- uphold and enhance the good reputation of the professions.

1.3   You are personally accountable for your practice. This means that you are answerable for your actions and omissions, regardless of advice or directions from another professional.

1.4   You have a duty of care to your patients and clients, who are entitled to receive safe and competent care.

1.5   You must adhere to the laws of the country in which you are practising.

2   As a registered nurse, midwife or specialist community public health nurse, you must respect the patient or client as an individual

2.1   You must recognise and respect the role of patients and clients as partners in their care and the contribution they can make to it. This involves identifying their preferences regarding care and respecting these within the limits of professional practice, existing legislation, resources and the goals of the therapeutic relationship.

2.2   You are personally accountable for ensuring that you promote and protect the interests and dignity of patients and clients, irrespective of gender, age, race, ability, sexuality, economic status, lifestyle, culture and religious or political beliefs.

2.3   You must, at all times, maintain appropriate professional boundaries in the relationships you have with patients and clients. You must ensure that all aspects of the relationship focus exclusively upon the needs of the patient or client.

2.4   You must promote the interests of patients and clients. This includes helping individuals and groups gain access to health and social care, information and support relevant to their needs.

2.5   You must report to a relevant person or authority, at the earliest possible time, any conscientious objection that may be relevant to your professional practice. You must continue to provide care to the best of your ability until alternative arrangements are implemented.

3   As a registered nurse, midwife or specialist community public health nurse, you must obtain consent before you give any treatment or care

3.1   All patients and clients have a right to receive information about their condition. You must be sensitive to their needs and respect the wishes of those who refuse or are unable to receive information about their condition. Information should be accurate, truthful and presented in such a way as to make it easily understood. You may need to seek legal or professional advice or guidance from your employer, in relation to the giving or withholding of consent.

3.2   You must respect patients' and clients' autonomy – their right to decide whether or not to undergo any health care intervention – even where a refusal may result in harm or death to themselves or a fetus, unless a court of law orders to the contrary. This right is protected in law, although in circumstances where the health of the fetus would be severely compromised by any refusal to give consent, it would be appropriate to discuss this matter fully within the team and with a supervisor of midwives, and possibly to seek external advice and guidance (see clause 4).

3.3   When obtaining valid consent, you must be sure that it is:
- given by a legally competent person
- given voluntarily
- informed.

3.4   You should presume that every patient and client is legally competent unless otherwise assessed by a suitably qualified practitioner. A patient or client who is legally competent can understand and retain treatment information and can use it to make an informed choice.

3.5   Those who are legally competent may give consent in writing, orally or by co-operation. They may also refuse consent. You must ensure that all your discussions and associated decisions relating to obtaining consent are documented in the patient's or client's health care records.

3.6   When patients or clients are no longer legally competent and have lost the capacity to consent to or refuse treatment and care, you should try to find out whether they have previously indicated preferences in an advance statement. You must respect any refusal of treatment or care given when they were legally competent, provided that the decision is clearly applicable to the present circumstances and that there is no reason to believe that they have changed their minds. When such a statement is not available, the patients' or clients' wishes, if known, should be taken into account. If these wishes are not known, the criteria for treatment must be that it is in their best interests.

3.7   The principles of obtaining consent apply equally to those people who have a mental illness. Whilst you should be involved in their assessment, it will also be necessary to involve relevant people close to them; this may include a psychiatrist. When patients and clients are detained under statutory powers (mental health acts), you must ensure that you know the circumstances and safeguards needed for providing treatment and care without consent.

3.8   In emergencies where treatment is necessary to preserve life, you may provide care without consent, if a patient or client is unable to give it, provided you can demonstrate that you are acting in their best interests.

3.9   No-one has the right to give consent on behalf of another competent adult. In relation to obtaining consent for a child, the involvement of those with parental responsibility in the consent procedure is usually necessary, but will depend on the age and understanding of the child. If the child is under the age of 16 in England and Wales, 12 in Scotland and 17 in Northern Ireland, you must be aware of legislation and local protocols relating to consent.

3.10   Usually the individual performing a procedure should be the person to obtain the patient's or client's consent. In certain circumstances, you may seek consent on behalf of colleagues if you have been specially trained for that specific area of practice.

3.11   You must ensure that the use of complementary or alternative therapies is safe and in the interests of patients and clients. This must be discussed with the team as part of the therapeutic process and the patient or client must consent to their use.

4   As a registered nurse, midwife or specialist community public health nurse, you must co-operate with others in the team

4.1   The team includes the patient or client, the patient's or client's family, informal carers and health and social care professionals in the National Health Service, independent and voluntary sectors.

4.2   You are expected to work co-operatively within teams and to respect the skills, expertise and contributions of your colleagues. You must treat them fairly and without discrimination.

4.3   You must communicate effectively and share your knowledge, skill and expertise with other members of the team as required for the benefit of patients and clients.

4.4   Health care records are a tool of communication within the team. You must ensure that the health care record for the patient or client is an accurate account of treatment, care planning and delivery. It should be consecutive, written with the involvement of the patient or client wherever practicable and completed as soon as possible after an event has occurred. It should provide clear evidence of the care planned, the decisions made, the care delivered and the information shared.

4.5   When working as a member of a team, you remain accountable for your professional conduct, any care you provide and any omission on your part.

4.6   You may be expected to delegate care delivery to others who are not registered nurses or midwives. Such delegation must not compromise existing care but must be directed to meeting the needs and serving the interests of patients and clients. You remain accountable for the appropriateness of the delegation, for ensuring that the person who does the work is able to do it and that adequate supervision or support is provided.

4.7   You have a duty to co-operate with internal and external investigations.

5   As a registered nurse, midwife or specialist community public health nurse, you must protect confidential information

5.1   You must treat information about patients and clients as confidential and use it only for the purposes for which it was given. As it is impractical to obtain consent every time you need to share information with others, you should ensure that patients and clients understand that some information may be made available to other members of the team involved in the delivery of care. You must guard against breaches of confidentiality by protecting information from improper disclosure at all times.

5.2   You should seek patients' and clients' wishes regarding the sharing of information with their family and others. When a patient or client is considered incapable of giving permission, you should consult relevant colleagues.

5.3   If you are required to disclose information outside the team that will have personal consequences for patients or clients, you must obtain their consent. If the patient or client withholds consent, or if consent cannot be obtained for whatever reason, disclosures may be made only where:
- they can be justified in the public interest (usually where disclosure is essential to protect the patient or client or someone else from the risk of significant harm)
- they are required by law or by order of a court.

5.4   Where there is an issue of child protection, you must act at all times in accordance with national and local policies.

6 As a registered nurse, midwife or specialist community public health nurse, you must maintain your professional knowledge and competence

6.1 You must keep your knowledge and skills up-to-date throughout your working life. In particular, you should take part regularly in learning activities that develop your competence and performance.

6.2 To practise competently, you must possess the knowledge, skills and abilities required for lawful, safe and effective practice without direct supervision. You must acknowledge the limits of your professional competence and only undertake practice and accept responsibilities for those activities in which you are competent.

6.3 If an aspect of practice is beyond your level of competence or outside your area of registration, you must obtain help and supervision from a competent practitioner until you and your employer consider that you have acquired the requisite knowledge and skill.

6.4 You have a duty to facilitate students of nursing, midwifery and specialist community public health nursing and others to develop their competence.

6.5 You have a responsibility to deliver care based on current evidence, best practice and, where applicable, validated research when it is available.

7 As a registered nurse, midwife or specialist community public health nurse, you must be trustworthy

7.1 You must behave in a way that upholds the reputation of the professions. Behaviour that compromises this reputation may call your registration into question even if is not directly connected to your professional practice.

7.2 You must ensure that your registration status is not used in the promotion of commercial products or services, declare any financial or other interests in relevant organisations providing such goods or services and ensure that your professional judgement is not influenced by any commercial considerations.

7.3 When providing advice regarding any product or service relating to your professional role or area of practice, you must be aware of the risk that, on account of your professional title or qualification, you could be perceived by the patient or client as endorsing the product. You should fully explain the advantages and disadvantages of alternative products so that the patient or client can make an informed choice. Where you recommend a specific product, you must ensure that your advice is based on evidence and is not for your own commercial gain.

7.4 You must refuse any gift, favour or hospitality that might be interpreted, now or in the future, as an attempt to obtain preferential consideration.

7.5 You must neither ask for nor accept loans from patients, clients or their relatives and friends.

8 As a registered nurse, midwife or specialist community public health nurse, you must act to identify and minimise the risk to patients and clients

8.1 You must work with other members of the team to promote health care environments that are conducive to safe, therapeutic and ethical practice.

8.2 You must act quickly to protect patients and clients from risk if you have good reason to believe that you or a colleague, from your own or another profession, may not be fit to practise for reasons of conduct, health or competence. You should be aware of the terms of legislation that offer protection for people who raise concerns about health and safety issues.

8.3 Where you cannot remedy circumstances in the environment of care that could jeopardise standards of practice, you must report them to a senior person with sufficient authority to manage them and also, in the case of midwifery, to the supervisor of midwives. This must be supported by a written record.

8.4 When working as a manager, you have a duty toward patients and clients, colleagues, the wider community and the organisation in which you and your colleagues work. When facing professional dilemmas, your first consideration in all activities must be the interests and safety of patients and clients.

8.5 In an emergency, in or outside the work setting, you have a professional duty to provide care. The care provided would be judged against what could reasonably be expected from someone with your knowledge, skills and abilities when placed in those particular circumstances.

9   Indemnity insurance

9.1 The NMC recommends that a registered nurse, midwife or specialist community public health nurse, in advising, treating and caring for patients/clients, has professional indemnity insurance. This is in the interests of clients, patients and registrants in the event of claims of professional negligence.

9.2 Some employers accept vicarious liability for the negligent acts and/or omissions of their employees. Such cover does not normally extend to activities undertaken outside the registrant's employment. Independent practice would not normally be covered by vicarious liability, while agency work may not. It is the individual registrant's responsibility to establish their insurance status and take appropriate action.

9.3 In situations where employers do not accept vicarious liability, the NMC recommends that registrants obtain adequate professional indemnity insurance. If unable to secure professional indemnity insurance, a registrant will need to demonstrate that all their clients/patients are fully informed of this fact and the implications this might have in the event of a claim for professional negligence.

Glossary

Accountable	Responsible for something or to someone.
Care	To provide help or comfort.
Competent	Possessing the skills and abilities required for lawful, safe and effective professional practice without direct supervision.
Patient and client	Any individual or group using a health service.
Reasonable	The case of Bolam v Friern Hospital Management Committee (1957) produced the following definition of what is reasonable. "The test is the standard of the ordinary skilled man exercising and professing to have that special skill. A man need not possess the highest expert skill at the risk of being found negligent... it is sufficient if he exercises the skill of an ordinary man exercising that particular art." This definition is supported and clarified by the case of Bolitho v City and Hackney Health Authority (1993).

Summary

As a registered nurse, midwife or specialist community public health nurse, you must:

- respect the patient or client as an individual
- obtain consent before you give any treatment or care
- co-operate with others in the team
- protect confidential information
- maintain your professional knowledge and competence
- be trustworthy
- act to identify and minimise the risk to patients and clients.

FURTHER INFORMATION

The *NMC code of professional conduct: standards for conduct, performance and ethics* is available on the Nursing and Midwifery Council's website at www.nmc-uk.org. Printed copies can be obtained by writing to the Publications Department, Nursing and Midwifery Council, 23 Portland Place, London W1B 1PZ, by fax on 020 7436 2924 or by e-mail at publications@nmc-uk.org.

A wide range of NMC standards and guidance publications expand upon and develop many of the professional issues and themes identified in *The NMC code of professional conduct: standards for conduct, performance and ethics.* All are available on the NMC's website. A list of current NMC publications is available either on the website or on request from the Publications Department as above.

Enquiries about the issues addressed in *The NMC code of professional conduct: standards for conduct, performance and ethics* should be directed in the first instance to the NMC's professional advice service at the address above, by e-mail at advice@nmc-uk.org, by telephone on 020 7333 6541/6550/6553 or by fax on 020 7333 6538.

The Nursing and Midwifery Council will keep *The NMC code of professional conduct: standards for conduct, performance and ethics* under review and any comments, suggestions or requests for further clarification are welcome, both from practitioners and members of the public. These should be addressed to the Director of Registration and Standards, NMC, 23 Portland Place, London W1B 1PZ.

November 2004

Appendix 3

An NMC Guide for Students of Nursing and Midwifery

Protecting the public through professional standards

As a pre-registration student of nursing or midwifery, you will already have started to think about your future career as a registered nurse or midwife. Once you have successfully completed your programme of education, you will need to register with the Nursing and Midwifery Council [NMC] before you can practise as a nurse or midwife. This leaflet sets out some basic information about the NMC and some guidance for the clinical experience you will undertake during your studies. It is based upon extensive consultation with individual pre-registration students of nursing and midwifery, organisations representing students and lecturers in higher education. The leaflet should be read in conjunction with advice provided by your higher education institution.

What does the NMC do?

The NMC is the regulatory body for nursing and midwifery. Our purpose is to establish and improve standards of nursing and midwifery care in order to protect the public. These standards are set out in the *Code of professional conduct*, which the NMC will send to you when you first register. We urge you to get hold of a copy now. You should be able to obtain it through your university; if not, please write to our Publications Department.

You may not be aware that the standards set by the NMC already apply to you. The level of entry to the programme of education that you are undertaking and the content, type and length of your programme are all part of these standards. Our other key tasks are to:

- maintain a register of qualified nurses and midwives
- set standards for nursing and midwifery education, practice and conduct
- provide advice for nurses and midwives on professional standards
- consider allegations of misconduct or unfitness to practise due to ill health.

Registration and professional accountability

When you successfully complete your course, your higher education institution will notify the NMC that you have met the required standards and that you are eligible for entry on the register. Your course director will also complete a declaration of good character form on your behalf. When we have received this information and you have paid your registration fee, your name will be entered on the NMC register and you will be eligible to practise as a registered practitioner.

Registration is not simply an administrative process. The NMC's register is an instrument of public protection and anyone can check the registered status of a nurse or midwife. Registering with the NMC demonstrates that you have met the standards expected of registered nurses and midwives. It also demonstrates that you are professionally accountable at all times for your acts and omissions.

Professional accountability involves weighing up the interests of patients, using your professional judgement and skills to make a decision and enabling you to account for the decision you make. On rare occasions, nurses and midwives fall short of the professional standards expected of them. The NMC investigates in the public interest any complaints made about the professional conduct or fitness to practise of registered nurses and midwives.

Throughout your career, you will need to keep up to date with developments in your area of practice. Your continuing professional development is an integral part of your professional accountability. In order to continue to practise, you will need to meet the NMC's standards for post-registration education and practice [PREP].

Detailed information about PREP is available in *The PREP Handbook*, which you can obtain free of charge by writing to the Publications Department. You will also need to complete a notification of practice form and pay your periodic registration fee when you renew your registration every three years. Practising midwives also need to complete a notification of intention to practise form annually.

GUIDANCE ON CLINICAL EXPERIENCE FOR STUDENTS

> During your studentship, you will come into close contact with patients. This may be through observing care being given, through helping in providing care and, later, through full participation in providing care. At all times, you should work only within your level of understanding and competence and always under the direct supervision of a registered nurse or midwife. The section below provides some guidance on working with patients during your studies. The principles underpinning this guidance reflect the standards that will be expected of you when you become a registered practitioner.

Your accountability

As a pre-registration student, you are **never** professionally accountable in the way that you will be after you come to register with the NMC. This means that you cannot be called to account for your actions and omissions by the NMC. So far as the NMC is concerned, it is the registered practitioners with whom you are working who are professionally responsible for the consequences of your actions and omissions. This is why you must always work under the direct supervision of a registered nurse or midwife. This does not mean, however, that you can never be called to account by your university or by the law for the consequences of your actions or omissions as a pre-registration student.

The wishes of patients

You must respect the wishes of patients at all times. They have the right to refuse to allow you, as a student, to participate in caring for them and you should make this right clear to them when they are first given information about the care they will receive from you. You should leave if they ask you to do so. Their rights as patients supersede at all times your rights to knowledge and experience.

Identifying yourself

Introduce yourself accurately at all times when speaking to patients either directly or by telephone. In doing so, you should make it quite clear that you are a pre-registration student and not a registered practitioner. In fact, it is a criminal offence to represent yourself falsely and deliberately as a registered nurse or midwife.

Accepting appropriate responsibility

You will find yourself at times in a position where you may not be directly accompanied by your mentor, supervisor or another registered colleague. You will also experience emergencies. As your skills, experience and confidence develop, you will become increasingly able to deal with these situations. However, as a student, do not participate in any procedure for which you have not been fully prepared or in which you are not adequately supervised. If such a situation arises, discuss the matter as quickly as possible with your supervisor.

Patient confidentiality

Patients have the right to know that any private and personal information that is given in confidence will be used only for the purposes for which it was originally provided and that it will not be used for any other reason. If you want to refer in a written assignment to some real-life situation in which you have been involved, do not provide any information that could identify a particular patient. Obtain access to patient records only when absolutely necessary for the care being provided. Use of these records must be closely supervised by a registered practitioner and you must follow the local policy on the handling and storage of records. Any written entry you make in a patient's records must be counter-signed by a registered practitioner. You can find more advice about confidentiality in the NMC's *Code of professional conduct*. You should also refer to our *Guidelines for records and record keeping*.

Handling complaints

Be aware of the local procedures for dealing with complaints by patients, or their families, about the treatment or care they are receiving. If patients indicate to you that they are unhappy about their treatment or care, you should report the matter immediately to the person who is supervising your clinical experience or to another appropriate person.

We hope that you will find these notes helpful during your studentship and in understanding the important responsibilities you will undertake as a registered nurse or midwife. If you need to discuss any of these issues with us, please contact our professional advice service on 020 7333 6541/6550/6553, by e-mail at advice@nmc-uk.org or by fax on 020 7333 6538. If you would like to find out more about the work of the NMC, please write to our Publications Department for a list of current publications. The NMC's website at www.nmc-uk.org includes copies of all NMC publications, position statements issued by our professional advice service and further useful information and contacts for students of nursing and midwifery. We wish you success in your programme of preparation for registration and in your future career.

Appendix 4
A Framework for Capable Practice

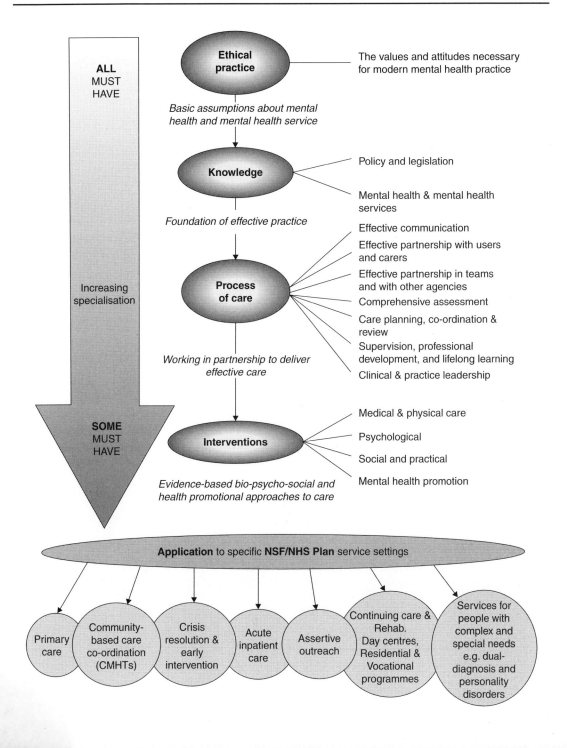

Ethical practice — The values and attitudes necessary for modern mental health practice

Basic assumptions about mental health and mental health service

Knowledge — Policy and legislation / Mental health & mental health services

Foundation of effective practice

Process of care — Effective communication / Effective partnership with users and carers / Effective partnership in teams and with other agencies / Comprehensive assessment / Care planning, co-ordination & review / Supervision, professional development, and lifelong learning / Clinical & practice leadership

Working in partnership to deliver effective care

Interventions — Medical & physical care / Psychological / Social and practical / Mental health promotion

Evidence-based bio-psycho-social and health promotional approaches to care

ALL MUST HAVE — Increasing specialisation — **SOME MUST HAVE**

Application to specific **NSF/NHS Plan** service settings

Primary care • Community-based care co-ordination (CMHTs) • Crisis resolution & early intervention • Acute inpatient care • Assertive outreach • Continuing care & Rehab. Day centres, Residential & Vocational programmes • Services for people with complex and special needs e.g. dual-diagnosis and personality disorders

Index

Numbers in **bold** refer to figures and tables.

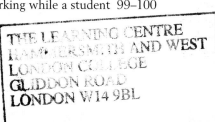

Midwife

To be a midwife, you need to have a friendly, gentle approach, be mindful of individual women's needs and respect their cultures. You need to always have the woman's wishes at heart, especially where she has a birth plan.

Skills Excellent people skills & Having babies happens to all sorts of people, so you will be providing professional support and reassurance to a huge diversity of women, during some of the most emotionally intense periods in their lives. Good communication and observation:-
Working as a midwife you will need to have an in-depth understanding of foetal and child development. It is also kept to update knowledge and ability to answer their questions.

Dealing with emotionally charged situations: Stay calm & alert in times of stress, and enable women to feel confident and in control.